Osteopathy Without Borders

Graham Mason

Grosvenor House
Publishing Limited

This book is published by
Grosvenor House Publishing Ltd
Link House
140 The Broadway, Tolworth, Surrey, KT6 7HT.
www.grosvenorhousepublishing.co.uk

A CIP record for this book
is available from the British Library

ISBN 978-1-80381-042-3

Table of Contents

This book is dedicated to my wife Jackie and my family who have given me great support over the years and especially to my granddaughter Hannah who has been invaluable in getting this book published.

Preface

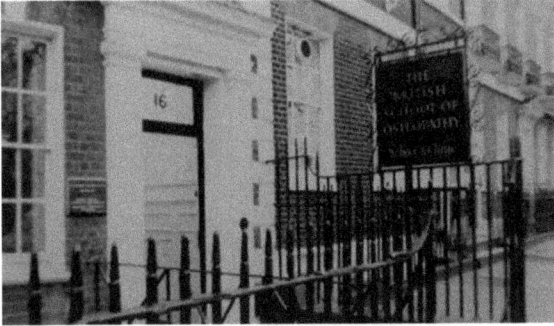

Where it all began – 16 Buckingham Gate London SW1.

I qualified at the British School of Osteopathy in 1966.

That year, twenty-four of us qualified and I joined what was then the registering body, The General Council and Register of Osteopaths [GCRO]. My certificate bore the number 400, so I was the 400th osteopath to be elected to the GCRO.

Since then I have been in private practice and have lectured throughout my career both in the UK and abroad.

During the 1980's and 90's I was part of a team that took the Osteopaths Act of 1993 through parliament.

I have always felt that osteopathic medicine has a large part to play in health care and gaining statutory regulation has placed osteopathy and osteopathic education in its rightful place in the medical jigsaw.

Prior to the Osteopaths Act there were over thirteen schools of osteopathy plus numerous apprenticeships. This was not good for the profession as there were no set standards of education. The Act ensured the highest educational standards in the osteopathic educational establishments and that we became a statutory regulated profession. Our profession was the first to be so regulated since the Dentists Act of 1922.

Now there are just five schools regulated by government through the General Osteopathic Council (GOsC) each offering a four-year course resulting in an integrated master's degree.

When I retired from everyday practice, I was asked what I was going to miss.

I replied that I would miss the differential diagnosis which is such an important part of an osteopath's life and I would miss treating babies and children.

When you palpate a neonate what you feel is unique.

However, I have been fortunate to continue lecturing both in the UK and abroad as I have been for many years.

I would like to thank all the students over the years who have given me the inspiration to carry on teaching and lecturing, for their enthusiasm and the questions they ask which have continued to make me think and self-reflect and understand my subject in a better way.

To the European School of Osteopathy, where I have taught for many years, a big thank you. Especially to those who have worked with me and to the staff and management team under the direction of the CEO Ian Fraser who have taken the school to the forefront of osteopathic education. It is, in my opinion, the only osteopathic teaching school to deliver a course that not only follows A.T. Still's philosophy but has brought it into the twenty-first century.

I am very grateful for all the support of my family, particularly my granddaughters, Chloe for letting me use her picture and Hannah for proofreading a lot of the chapters, getting the book proof read and helping me develop this book.

Also, to Hilary Percival, Andrew and Inga Allen and to Michelle Miller for their comments and support.

My thanks also go to Inga Allen for letting me to use baby Eli as a model in the paediatric chapter and to Inga, Cecile Keiner and Claudia Knox for helping with the paediatric chapter.

Finally, I would like to thank my friends Professor Frank Willard of the University of New England who I have worked and lectured with for many years and from whom I have learnt so much, and Dr Jane Carreiro, Dean of the New England College of Osteopathic Medicine, for her help over the years and to both of them for allowing me to use their wonderful dissection pictures.

CHAPTER 1

Prologue

"There is a tide in the affairs of men which, taken at the flood, leads on to fortune. Omitted, all the voyage of their life is bound in the shallows and in miseries. On such a sea are we now afloat and we must take the current when it serves. Or lose our ventures."

William Shakespeare, Julius Caesar Act IV

The French have a word, "transmettre", with its sense of "to hand over" something passed between eras. In this book I want to pass on what I have learnt over the past fifty-five years in osteopathy. I want others to see it clearly in all its strange beauty.

It is my firm belief that we must pass our knowledge on to the next generation or we will fail them.

Movement, shape and form is totally fascinating and no more so than in vertebrates and especially the human being.

It is the interrelationship of structures and how this has evolved that I find so interesting. From conception, as the human form develops in utero, cells divide and multiply and this human form is laid out systematically. A preordained geometry, so that all our working parts are somatically, neurologically and viscerally interrelated.

I hope this book will be of use to students and practitioners in osteopathy who wish to use the involuntary mechanism (IVM) and the primary respiratory mechanism (PRM) and for those, who, having learnt something of the involuntary mechanics, wish to learn more. To explore and increase their knowledge in this field, which will take them into another world; that of interrelated structures and treating the whole person.

1

In writing this book I am giving my view of osteopathic medicine, that I have gained in over fifty-five years in the profession. Having qualified at the British School of Osteopathy in Buckingham Gate in 1966, I entered into an assistantship with Colin Dove who had qualified ten years earlier, I was his first associate.

For the first few years my treatments were classical osteopathy, having been taught by some brilliant teachers such as Keith Blagrave (Peter Blagraves' father), Clem Middleton, Shenton Webster Jones, Audrey Smith and many others. At one point in our final year we were given talks by osteopaths who had been in practice some considerable time.

One of them came down from Preston in Lancashire. He explained that he had been seeing patients that morning and that they were a mixed bag of cases. One of my fellow students asked him what sort of conditions he had treated, expecting to be told about low back pain, sciatica and shoulder problems.

"Well" he said "I saw two cases of bronchitis and two patients with bad heart problems and one of tonsillitis."

I was spellbound. Here was someone who did not just massage and click joints. Here was a man treating conditions that we had only read about in text books so we could be good diagnosticians and pass our final exams.

After a few years in practice I was reflecting on what he had said in my final year as a student, and thinking about going with my grandmother, a large French lady, who regularly went to an osteopath in Stoke Newington London, a Dr Raby who qualified in America. I used to watch him treat her. She did not take her clothes off and he would pull her around in all sorts of ways to, in his words, "get the body to work for itself" and at a young age I thought no more of it until now

Something was lacking in my osteopathic world.

Colin Dove being an inquisitive person began to explore the IVM that some called cranial osteopathy and with the encouragement of Joyce Vetterlein who worked with me, I went on my first cranial course in London, run by the American osteopath Edna Ley. Edna had worked with Sutherland, Fulford and Becker. She was a colleague of Ann Wales and had a no-nonsense approach to teaching the IVM.

It was an epiphany. I came away both invigorated and confused. In one sense I had palpated things that I did not know existed but on the other hand I could not fathom out how it worked. Also, when working I had to have complete silence, as any interruption I lost where I was palpating.

Gradually this improved and I became sufficiently confident to embark on a course, which would become one of many, in the United States where I learned not only how the involuntary mechanism worked but how effective it could be.

I went to the University of New England and there I met some amazing osteopathic teachers and practitioners.

One of them was a man called John Harakall. Although he worked primarily with the IVM, he involved other classical techniques when he thought this was appropriate.

I arrived in class having flown in the day before. At these lectures there was one teacher to four students. I tried to work, but John said "you are jet-lagged, here, lie down and I will treat you."

He was going to treat me using the IVM however, he said "I can't do this, everything is solid." He stood up and immediately used High velocity technique (HVT) (dog technique) then sat at my head again and when he put his hands on, he said "that is better, everything is breathing."

This was a revelation to me because previously I had been advised by those who were working with the IVM that you could not combine the two methods of treatment. There was no rational explanation and working with John Harakall made me realise that there was no real differentiation as it is all osteopathy. It was all about movement; from minute cellular movement to the gross

3

movement of big muscles, and you used of your hands to bring about change, relief and healing.

As osteopaths we have to be self-reflective. We have to continue to learn, and failure is something that all osteopaths must understand, whether it is the failure to communicate or the failure to reach the correct diagnosis. Failure is a learning experience. It teaches you humility. It teaches you to work harder and it is a powerful motivator.

As one lecturer said to us, "you are only as good as the next patient – the last one was history."

To get the most out of osteopathy you cannot be narrow-minded, you have to think globally and tangentially. In other words, you have to think in all dimensions.

In this book I will concentrate on the IVM. The term cranial osteopathy, which is often applied, is a misnomer, as the expression we feel can be felt all over the body.

Practitioners who work with the IVM realise that osteopathic manipulative medicine (OMM) is treating the whole person, not what is thought of in some quarters as simply an effective treatment option for back pain and musculoskeletal disorders, an adjunct to minor orthopaedics. Andrew Taylor Still realised that changes in the anatomical system could have far-reaching effects within the rest of the body.

The globally-thinking osteopath has to include the psyche, the viscera and the soma (the musculoskeletal system), knowing that they are inextricably linked, and that changes in one of these areas will automatically affect the other two.

You have to consider the role of viscero-somatic reflexes and how the psyche can affect the rest of the body.

William Garner Sutherland (W G S) was a student of Dr Stills and a man with vision, energy and an enquiring mind.

William Sutherland took his vision of moveable bones in the cranium into a therapeutic concept.

4

He states, "I had to perform many serious experiments on my own cranium because of my scepticism about the mobility of the cranial bones. I could not perform these experiments on the heads of other people. However, I did need to perform them on a living head because it was to have the knowledge that is unobtainable from the study of a dead specimen in an anatomical laboratory. Had I tried them on another person I would have only have had information: they would have the knowledge."

I am sure that all osteopaths who begin to study the involuntary mechanism have a scepticism; virtually every student I have taught has been sceptical at first. This is healthy, for you are asking deep questions and not just accepting things in blind faith.

There are a lot of unanswered questions.

The manipulative medicine approach as a whole is still being questioned for its efficacy. Even very recently the beneficial effects of the short and long-term osteopathic manipulative medicine (OMM) has come into question. However, those practising OMM know from their own outcome studies that it is effective including those using the involuntary mechanism.

Nelson [2] et al. in 2006 wrote; "the techniques associated with treatment in the cranial field are possibly most controversial form of osteopathic medicine."

There have been studies, by Fryman (1971) osteopathic treatment of children: Tettambell (1978 and 2004) who compared osteopathic treatment in postnatal care: Rogers and Witt (1997) and Upledger and (2003) all examined the palpation of the IVM especially comparing the movement between the head and the feet.

In 1987 Feinberg and Mark examined the movement of the brain and cerebrospinal fluid confirming the existence of movement.

As early as 1865, Ludwig Traube found that there was rhythmic variation in blood pressure usually extending over several respiratory cycles, with a frequency varying from 6-10 cycles per minute, which related to variations in vasomotor tone. Ewald Hering confirmed this in 1869 and Siegmund Mayer observed similar oscillations in 1876.

According to Nelson et al. (JAOA 2001) these phenomena, known collectively as the Traube-Hering-Meyer (THM) oscillation, have been measured in association with heart rate, blood pressure, cardiac contractibility, pulmonary blood flow, cerebral blood flow, movement of the cerebrospinal fluid (CSF) and peripheral blood flow. This whole-body phenomenon, which exhibits a rate slightly less than independent respiration, bears a striking resemblance to what we as osteopaths understand as the primary respiratory mechanism (PRM).

In their detailed study, published in March 2001, they concluded that, "The THM oscillation may well represent one aspect of the complex clinical area of Sutherland's discovery. It may explain the rate and rhythm of the cranial rhythmical impulse (CRI) and offer an insight into the physiologic mechanism of the PRM and it may represent a component of the inherent mobility of the central nervous system (CNS)."

In some areas circulatory and body core temperature homeostasis are considered to be a result of the THM oscillation.

Magoun in Osteopathy in the Cranial Field states that the PRM is a dynamic metabolic interchange in every cell with each phase of action. Ninety-nine per cent of interstitial fluid exists in a gel-like state demonstrating some elasticity.

Those of us who work with the involuntary mechanism know the therapeutic effects that working with it can have, although in some instances we do not know via the pathway of research, how it works. However, if you know your anatomy, applied anatomy and have a deep knowledge of the interrelationship of structures, you know that you can have an effect on areas far removed from where you are palpating.

Elizabeth Hayden in the magazine Osteopathy Today, November 2011, states, "By applying a detailed knowledge of anatomy to your palpation, three-dimensional anatomy comes to life."

As osteopaths we are working with the interrelationship of structures but this does not just rest with the anatomy of the musculoskeletal system.

The more I work with the IVM I realise that we are working with low pressure fluid systems, interstitial fluid, intra and intercellular fluid, the fascia which is also a fluid, and that sometimes unquantifiable thing call potency (potency is defined as having the inherent capacity for growth and development.)

Handoll, in his book Anatomy of Potency, states, "The motion of the primary respiratory mechanism is not the potency. The motion is the expression of the potency. The potency is the desire, the potential, the need to express motion. The motion is acting out of the potency." That potency is expressed through fluid.

Sutherland states in Teachings in the science of osteopathy that our "knowledge is like that of an electrician who merely knows the potent current is present. It is learning how to stabilize that force that is important.

When working with the IVM I am looking at movement and lack of movement and motility. Improving it when restricted and restoring homeostasis."

By practice and perseverance, you can learn to identify different tissues such as hair, skin, fatty layers, bone, muscle, ligaments, fascia and fluid.

We are seventy per cent fluid and we can, with time and diligence, learn to feel different types of fluid from CSF to lymph and interstitial fluid and intercellular fluid.

Elizabeth Hayden states that "learning to palpate the rhythmic impulses of the involuntary mechanism feels as though the tissues are breathing."

Magoun and others have dealt with the cranial anatomy very well, but to understand it further it is imperative that you have a good understanding of the relevant applied anatomy.

In the next few chapters I am going to examine how we palpate and then look at the detailed anatomy and applied anatomy of the cranium and the face before looking detailed conditions and how to apply osteopathic techniques looking at the body as a whole.

There is one thing I must cover before I continue and that is development through the midline and that because we have a midline our body has two lateral equal parts. Osteopaths have embraced this concept of the midline. In IVM when the cranial base rises in the flexion phase, the paired structures externally rotate from the midline and in the extension phase the paired structures internally rotate.

The notochord is what all osteopaths working with the IVM know as our midline.

The notochord derives from the primitive node and is mesodermal. It is developed in the third week of intrauterine life and begins as the cranial midline extension from the primitive node of a hollow tube. This tube grows in length as primitive node cells are added to its proximal end as the primitive streak regresses.

On about day twenty the notochordal process is completely formed. It converts from a hollow tube to a flattened plate and then to a solid rod.

The notochord plays an important structural role. As a tissue, it is most closely related to cartilage and is likely to represent a primitive form of cartilage. Accordingly, the notochord serves as the axial skeleton of the embryo until other elements, such as the vertebrae, form.

During later development the rudiments of the vertebral bodies coalesce around the notochord, the midline.

CHAPTER 2

Palpation

Palpation is the art of feeling with one's hands, using the sense of touch. It is a skill the osteopath refines to a high degree.

When you first see your patient, you take a detailed case history. Then you observe. You look at the shape of the face, the contours of the body. Do they have a scoliosis? Is one shoulder higher than the other? Are the limbs symmetrical or is one arm or foot internally or externally rotated? You next carry out a physical examination.

You are building up a picture of how this body works.

But this is only part of the picture.

Next, place your hands on the patient. Feel the body, let the body talk to you, does the tissue under your hands feel tense or at ease? Is it soft and pliable or does the tissue feel irritable; is there vibrancy, does it feel tired?

You are allowing the body to tell you how it is working and by doing so you get a very good picture of the health of that person.

Before I give any treatment, I always let the body talk to me. There are so many different variants.

I remember treating one of my longstanding patients who had just had a mastectomy. The mechanism was very tired, it felt exhausted, there was no energy. It was as though the body had been drained of energy, which is not surprising when you think of what it had gone through, not just with the operation but the months preceding, the physical and mental changes that had been made. The wonderful thing about osteopathy is that you can help the body to repair, improve the energy, give the body back its life.

Holly was tiny a few weeks old. She was slightly premature at birth. She was seemingly lifeless. Sutherland, Ann Wales and

Rollin Becker all spoke about the spark of life, that amazing electrification/ the potency of the body that allows it to function.

When I put my hands-on Holly, I could not feel any movement, there was nothing, she just felt like a mass of protoplasm, dough-like, inert. Slowly I worked to find something, some movement, some change. I balanced the membrane around the sella turcica, I lifted the parietals to try to give space and then something happened. There was a swelling beneath my hands it was as though her whole body had taken a deep breath. There was life, there was an energy that was not there before.

In the weeks and months that followed she went from strength to strength, and although she had been slightly palsied, she has grown into a remarkable young lady, she is now in her late twenties. Her slight palsy is still there but she can drive, she can hold down a job and she is delightful company.

When palpating you have to feel between your hands, spatially. This will allow you to feel in depth and by practice and more practice you will develop a very sensitive palpatory skill.

If at any time you find that your palpation is such that you do not feel anything, or very little, do not be concerned as there are several reasons for this.

Firstly, the involuntary mechanism may just be quiet or maybe you are trying too hard to feel and this sometimes shuts the mechanism down.

As that amazing American osteopath Ann Wales always used to say "wait for the mechanism to talk to you, sometimes this can take a little while."

I remember her words vividly. "Let the mechanism talk to you."

I was treating my granddaughter. Sometimes it is not always easy to treat your own kin. Colleagues have often bought their new babies to see me because they do not find it easy to treat them.

However, this day I was treating Jade, aged twelve, who had been dancing for some time and had developed a painful hip.

I placed my hands on her with one hand under the hip joint and the other with a thumb on the greater tuberosity of the femur, my forearm resting along the femur, and my fingers spread out along the inguinal ligament. I had the whole hip and the rotators between my hands.

I waited and waited but could not feel a thing. I was waiting to palpate the flexion and extension phases where the femur would externally and internally rotate, once I was feeling it, I could balance the hip with its rotators. But nothing happened. Jade's mother was asking what was happening, when suddenly I began to feel the movement and my granddaughter looked up and said "you are in now."

Patience is sometimes a forgotten art when treating a patient.

So, firstly make sure that your stance is good. Sit well back in your chair and have your feet solidly on the ground. Let your shoulders and forearms relax with your elbows on the table forming good listening posts. Now make sure that you are not too intense in searching for the mechanism.

Try to think of your own straight sinus. Are you balanced?

If you are tense or feel unbalanced, without your patient knowing, have a deep yawn as this will relax all your facial and neck muscles and the diaphragm.

Your intensity and the temptation to search for the mechanism may easily slow it down or stop it all together. If this does happen try to imagine yourself standing behind yourself and looking on. In other words, "back off"; relax, think of the trees outside or as I often say to my students "get your mind in the car park." Once you do this then you will begin to feel. The more you relax your body and especially your hands the more you will feel.

In all the years I have taught the involuntary mechanism (IVM) I can count on the fingers of one hand the number of students who at the end of the course cannot palpate the mechanism.

Palpation is the skill of feeling different tissues and structures with your hands. With your fingers, the palm of your hand and the thenar and hypothenar areas. As you develop your skills you will be able to palpate with the forearms as they rest on the body.

Palpation is purely subjective and it is very easy, when in the early stages of learning, to imagine what you feel, either because you are told what you should feel or you have read it or you are just thinking about the anatomy. Do not be drawn into this trap. You have to feel in in layers

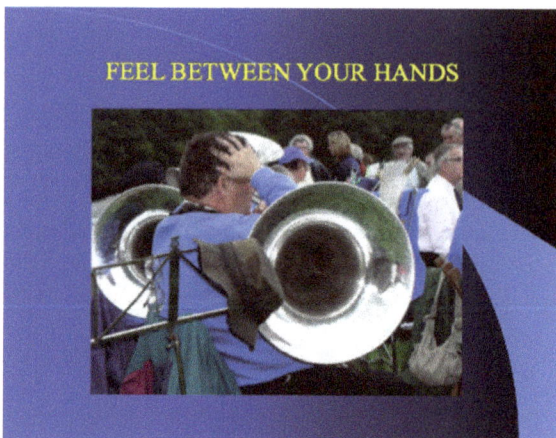

Feeling between your hands increases what you can feel;
it turns up the volume.

Palpation of the cranium should begin with feeling the hair, the skin and the fascia underlying it. By doing this you will then easily move on to the cranial bones. So, you will begin to feel in depth.

You have to use your hands as eyes, and you have a number of eyes. All your fingers, thumbs, also the thenar and hypothenar eminences. By working with the whole of your hand you will be able to palpate in three dimensions.

When you palpate the cranial bones remember that this is living tissue you are palpating; it has a blood supply, drainage and a soft diploe, it breathes.

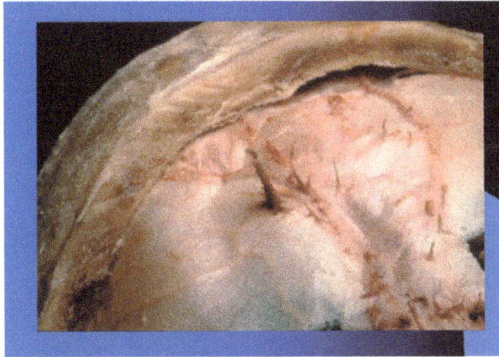

Dural membrane showing the blood supply to
the vault bones through the membrane.
Used with permission of the Willard/Carreiro Collection

Palpate the movement of the cranial bones in the respiratory
phases of flexion and extension. Remember in the flexion phase
the cranial base rises, the body becomes shorter and fatter and the
paired structures externally rotate. In the extension phase the
cranial base lowers and the body becomes longer and thinner and
the paired structures internally rotate.

Examine each bone in turn beginning with the parietals.
Palpate the mobility of these two bones and their axis of movement

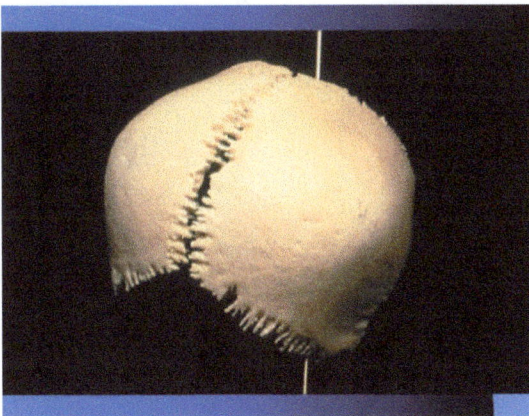

Note the axis of movement from anteromedial to posterolateral.
Used with permission of the Willard/Carreiro Collection

Note the change in the bevels of the sagittal suture. The bevels are tighter anteriorly and become wider the more posterior you go. This change in bevelling shows that there is a greater range of movement posteriorly than anteriorly.

Now palpate the frontal bones. Working with the IVM you must always consider the frontal as being two bones, for they begin life as two bones separated by the metopic suture.

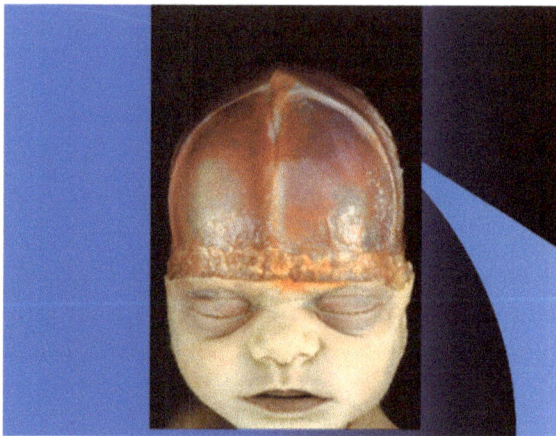

Neonate frontal bone, note the metopic suture.
Used with permission of the Willard/Carreiro Collection

Feel how the frontal bone moves. In the flexion phase it will move anteroinferiorly and externally rotate so that the sphenofrontal border will move anteriorly and laterally. Consider the relationship with the adjacent bones, the sphenoid, ethmoid, zygoma, nasal bones and the lacrimal bones. Especially consider the articulation with the parietal bones along the coronal suture and the changes in bevelling that occur from the medial to lateral aspect so that there is more movement laterally than medially.

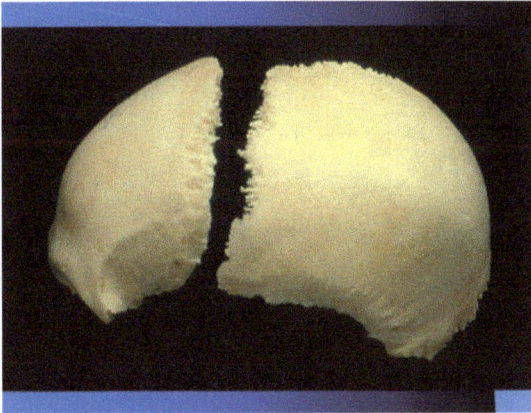

Observe carefully the change in the bevel of the coronal suture.
Used with permission of the Willard/Carreiro Collection

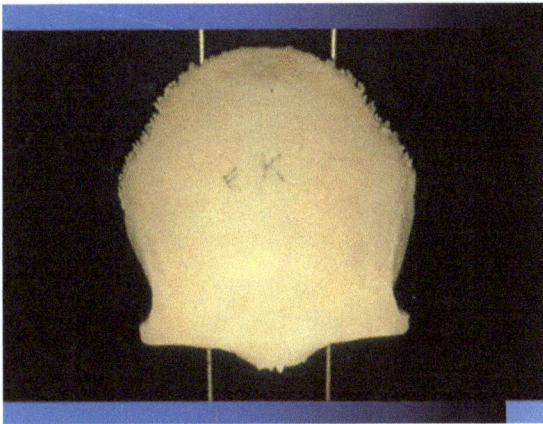

Axis of movement of the frontal bone.
Used with permission of the Willard/Carreiro Collection

By palpating the vault bones, you are building up a picture of how the involuntary mechanism is working.

But, remember you are palpating not treating. Over the years so many students, when they begin to palpate and find the mechanism instinctively, begin to treat, to change things.

CHAPTER 3

The Membrane

If you now go deeper in your palpation, still thinking between your hands, you will come to a structure that has a different feel to the bony structures. It has a different texture. Laterally it feels quite firm but if you follow it medially you will find it softer and more compliant.

This is the membrane and what you are feeling is the firm outer border surrounding the brain and medially you are palpating the tentorium cerebelli on its medial border.

The membrane is fascia and fascia is fluid. 30 per cent is intracellular, 35 per cent intravascular plus interstitial fluid.

It surrounds the brain and the neural tube and is attached to all the longitudinal ligaments as far as S2.

The membrane is a continuum of the outer layer, the dura mater; Latin for tough mother, the middle layer the arachnoid mater; Latin for spiderweb like, and the inner pia mater; Latin for tender mother.

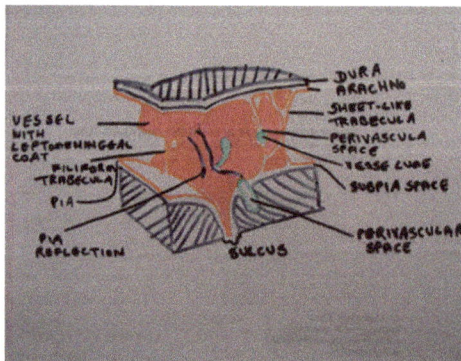

The continuum of the three layers of the membrane.

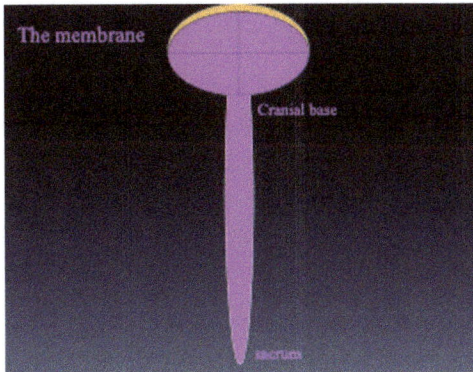

If you look at a dissected cadaver, the membrane has the texture of chicken skin. It is inelastic, but it allows movement.

The brain and the spinal cord are constantly changing shape due to their texture, fluidity and the changing fluid state.

The brain is surrounded by cerebrospinal fluid (CSF) contained within the membrane and the cisterns. This gives the brain buoyancy and protection.

The CSF is constantly being produced in the ventricles. The main production is via the choroid plexus in the lateral ventricles, the third and fourth ventricles where it exits through the foramen of Magendie.

There is about 125ml of CSF at any one time and it is produced at a rate of 350 micro litres per minute. Reabsorption is through the arachnoid granulations in the sagittal sinus although there is also natural weepage through the nerve exits and reabsorption also takes place through the lymphatic system.

The CSF occupies the subarachnoid space between the arachnoid mater and pia mater so therefore is an integral part of the membrane.

Remember that the membrane is a single unit completely surrounding the brain and the spinal cord and it is attached to the foramen magnum and to all the posterior longitudinal ligaments down to S2.

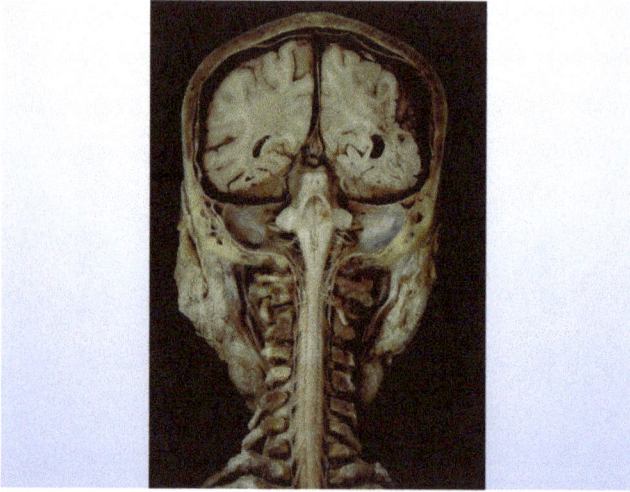

This picture shows the membrane surrounding the brain and exiting
through the foramen magnum. Notice also the midline falx cerebri
and the tentoria cerebelli beneath the cerebral hemispheres.
Used with permission of the Willard/Carreiro Collection

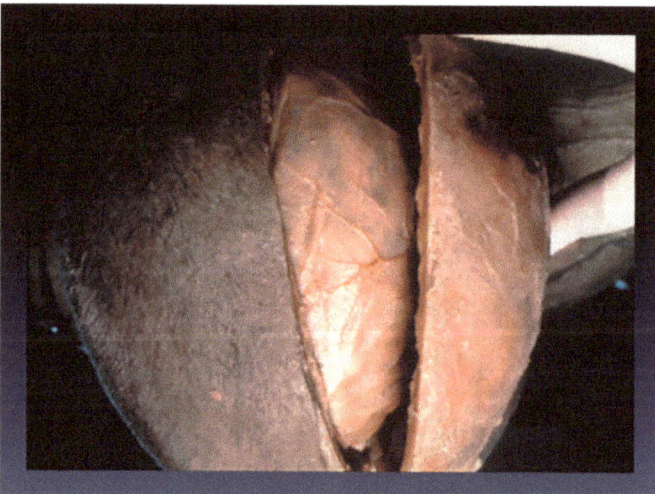

The bony calvarium opened showing the membrane.
Notice the blood supply.
Used with permission of the Willard/Carreiro Collection

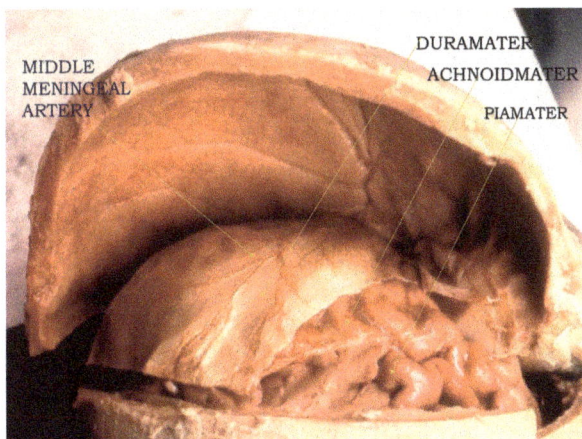

This slide shows the membrane as a continuum and
the blood supply of the middle meningeal artery.
Used with permission of the Willard/Carreiro Collection

To palpate the membrane via the cranium, take a simple vault hold. Have good listening posts and relax. Palpate the bony tissue. Then palpate a little more deeply, feel between your hands, and you will feel the membrane; it will feel very different to the bony tissue. Use your hands as eyes and "look" at its texture. Is it relaxed, tense, tight? Gain an overall impression as what you are feeling.

To improve your palpation, practise palpating the membrane. Feel the differences between the harder fixed part of the tentorium covering the bony skull and its softer free medial border.

Whilst you are palpating the membrane consider the sinuses that are held within it. This is especially important when palpating the falx cerebri. The superior sagittal sinus is housed in the superior aspect of the falx and drains the superior aspect of the vault; it also houses the arachnoid granulations through which CSF is reabsorbed through a simple gating mechanism.

The firm attachment of the lateral border of the tentorium to the bony tissue feels very different to the free-floating medial border. As an exercise follow the tentorium posteriorly to where it converges with the falx cerebri. Then follow the falx cerebri anteriorly until you eventually reach a much firmer point. This is the point where the falx cerebri is attached to the crista galli of the ethmoid bone. The membrane will then spread out laterally along the frontal bone and the lesser and greater wings of the sphenoid bone.

Now move your palpation posteriorly and you will reach the convergence of the tentorium and the falx cerebri. It is here that you will find the straight sinus leading slightly superiorly and anteriorly towards the ventricles. It is along this sinus, otherwise known to those who work with the involuntary movement as the Sutherland fulcrum, where a point of balance or a fulcrum can be found. This fulcrum can be anywhere along the straight sinus but more often than not it is within the middle third.

The definition of a fulcrum is [1] "a pivot that allows leverage or on which it turns or is supported. [2] A point of balance. From the Latin fulcire: to prop. The means by which influence is brought to bear."

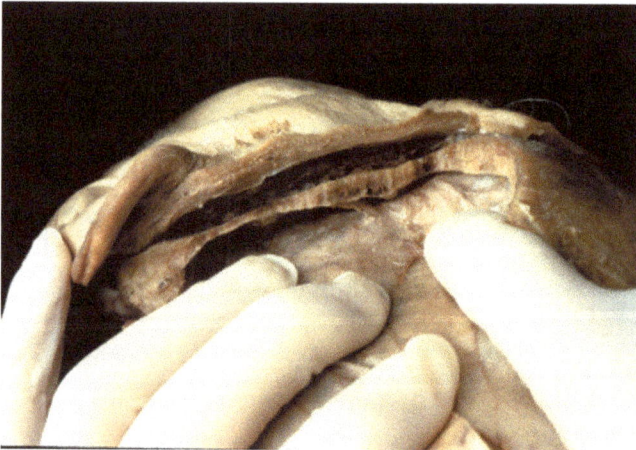

Remember the membrane is attached to the bony cranium.
Used with permission of the Willard/Carreiro Collection

Once you can palpate the falx cerebri and the tentorium you can move your palpation below the straight sinus onto the falx cerebri.

Anatomically the falx cerebelli descends from the inferior aspect of the straight sinus inferiorly and anteriorly to the attachment on the posterior aspect of the foramen magnum.

From this point you are able to palpate the membrane around the foramen magnum, and you can follow the membrane through the foramen magnum and caudally down the spinal dural tube. Palpate through the foramen try to see how far you can follow the dural tube caudally. Feel how different it feels in certain places, this will be due to facial changes or restrictions within the vertebral joints such as crush fractures and intervertebral discs that have spread laterally.

If, when palpating, you find that you have lost the firm texture of the membrane and your palpatory sense is lighter and far more mobile, then you are probably palpating the fluid (CSF) and should ease back in your palpation a little to be able to feel the delicate yet firm membrane.

Balanced membranous tension

Once you have palpated and examined the membrane you can consider taking it to a point of balance along the straight sinus otherwise known as the Sutherland fulcrum.

Place your hands in a vault hold but be careful not to allow your fingers to slip below the cranial base onto the upper cervical spine. If this does happen you may find yourself drawn down inferiorly along the cervical fascia.

Once you have engaged the membrane, find the straight sinus and if you examine it you will find a point along it where there is a fulcrum. This is a point where the planes of movement coincide.

Focus on this point. You will have the whole membrane in between your hands.

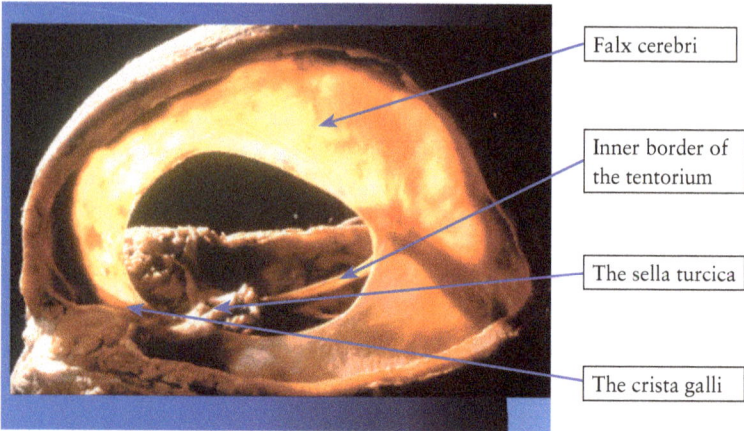

Fig 2 Showing the falx cerebri the tentorium showing free edges and the sella turcica and the attachment of the falx to the crista galli. Used with permission of the Willard/Carreiro Collection

Balancing the membrane along the Sutherland fulcrum is like trying to balance a ball in the centre of a drum skin.

When you have found a focal fulcrum, follow the movement in whichever direction it moves. Follow it to a point of ease, continue and gradually refine the movement. It will become less and less until you reach a point where you do not feel anything. You have now reached a point of balance.

However, *wait*, because the point of balance has a habit of moving very slightly, like a bird settling on a nest, and it can do this several times until it reaches a point where you will feel everything totally relax and become very still.

I liken it to looking into a black hole, there is no sensation of movement at all.

If you have ever been on top of a mountain there are times when you can feel, even touch the silence; the point of balance is like that, a blankness, nothing is happening.

Wait patiently; after a short while you will feel a soft but powerful movement that is more compliant. The mechanism is commencing another cycle.

Now you can decide at which point you can take your hands off.

Another method of balancing the membrane is to balance it around the diaphragm of sellae. The diaphragm of sellae is a membranous diaphragm over the sella turcica.

The sella turcica is a deep depression in the body of the sphenoid bone and which houses the pituitary gland. The pituitary stalk or infundibulum connects the pituitary gland to the hypothalamus.

This is the core of our midline.

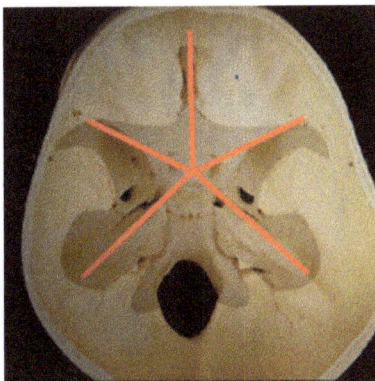

Taking a vault hold, the whole membrane can be palpated between your hands. You are looking to reach a point of balance in the middle of the sella turcica this will be your fulcrum, in the midline.

You use the same technique as above, following the movement in all directions until you refine it and it becomes less and less. You finally will reach a point where all the movement is refined around one point, the fulcrum, and here you will find appoint of balance, then stillness. As before it is like looking down a black hole, such is the stillness. Very soon you will find your hands feeling movement and a new cycle will begin.

I find this method allows you to obtain a much finer balance and you can feel it affecting the whole body at the same time.

Before we leave this chapter on the membrane, we must consider whiplash injuries because the membrane is always compromised in whiplash injuries.

GRAHAM MASON

Patients who have been involved in road traffic accidents or any other injury where the spine and cranium move forcibly and quickly in one direction present in our practices at regular intervals. Rugby football is a good example of how many more whiplash injuries we see due to the increase in a heavy blocking tackle.

Consider what is happening to the membrane during a whiplash incident and how it is affected. The diagram above shows how a whiplash injury can affect all the tissues with in the body.

Our bodies are seventy per cent fluid. When you knock over a container of fluid, the fluid will be pushed out of the container in the same direction as the force exerted on it. As you palpate the cranium you will be able to tell the direction of the force of impact that caused the whiplash, therefore with your palpatory skill you will be able to restore some form of normality.

Research has shown that the fulcrum for all whiplash injuries is the fifth cervical vertebra.

Kaneoka, Ono, Inami and Hayashi in their paper in Spine (April 1999) found that there were three distinct patterns of motion in the cervical spine after impact from a rear-end collision, culminating in C5-6 showing an open book motion with an upward-shifted instantaneous axis of movement.

Finally, we must remember that within this membrane there is a large complex of venous drainage as the diagram below shows. By working with the membrane, you can have a distinct effect on this venous drainage which is so important. Consider the sagittal sinus and the constant change of CSF and that this sinus needs space and movement to be able to operate efficiently. The sinuses all drain caudally. Eventually all the fluid will be transported by the internal jugular vein.

Remember there is a very large fluid exchange within the cranium, arterial, venous, lymphatic and extracellular fluid and CSF.

CHAPTER 4

The Face

All through life we are drawn to looking at a face. How many of us people-watch when in an airport or railway station? We look at the shape, the contours, the smile, the frown and build up an image of that person and their personality. Are they happy, angry, sad? Are they anxious? As with palpation, when you let the body talk to you, let the face talk to you also.

Does the face look comfortable, does it give the impression of working as a pump? Because in the end that is what the face does, the movement within the face helps and contrives to move fluid, whether it is sinus fluid, lymphatic fluid, venous or arterial fluid, interstitial fluid, intra and extracellular fluid, there is *always* fluid movement.

We observe osteopathically because that is how we are trained.

I remember Dr Melicien Tettambel, an American osteopath/obstetrician gynaecologist, saying that we osteopaths are interesting people, always observing.

She told a story of being in a shop and a lady came in with a new baby in a pram. All the people gathered round and were cooing over the child saying how pretty she was. "All I could think of" said Tetambell looking at the child was, "wow, what a side bending rotation".

A number of years ago an experiment was conducted where people of the opposite sex were shown videos of six people walking and sitting. They observed their gait, their face and their smile. The result showed that we are attracted to people by the shape of the face and different people are attracted to different faces. This is not so surprising except that osteopaths are attracted to the face for very different reasons.

To be able to treat the face and its associated structures successfully there has to be an understanding of the embryology. Only by understanding how the face develops can you begin to understand the interrelationship of the structures.

The face, the head and the neck are developed in a series of pharyngeal arches, pharyngeal pouches and grooves.

In evolutionary terms the pharyngeal arches are evolved from the gill arches of the jawless fishes and in jawed vertebrates. The first arch gives rise to the lower jaw or mandible.

These arches are formed very early on in intrauterine life, from approximately day 22 to day 30 in a craniocaudal sequence. The arches are numbered 1 to 6 although it is thought that arch 5 does not exist in humans or if it does it is very short-lived.

If you look closely at these arches, they consist of somitic mesoderm and neural crest cells and each one has a cranial nerve associated with it.

The mesoderm forms arteries and muscle, and the neural crest forms connective tissue, cartilage and bone.

By understanding the development and the structures involved with each arch you can have a much better understanding of the interrelationships, which will give you, as an osteopath, a deeper insight and be able to formulate a more effective treatment plan.

The first arch is the mandibular arch and it is associated with the trigeminal nerve, cranial nerve V, it is the largest cranial nerve. It is one third motor and two thirds sensory. The motor component supplies the muscles of mastication. The mylohyoid, the tensor veli palatini, tensor tympani and the anterior belly of the digastric muscle are all supplied by the trigeminal nerve. The sensory component is sensory to the face.

The maxilla, zygoma, palatine, vomer and the squamous part of the temporal bone as well as the incus, malleus, the mandible and the sphenomandibular ligament and the anterior ligament of the malleus are also derivatives of the first arch as is the maxillary artery.

The second pharyngeal arch is also known as the hyoid arch and is associated with cranial nerve VII, the facial nerve. As one would expect, the muscles of facial expression are also derived from the second arch as are the posterior belly of the digastric, stylohyoid and the stapedius muscles.

The other structures derived from the second pharyngeal arch are the upper part and the lesser horn of the hyoid bone, the stapes and the styloid process and ligament.

The third arch is associated with the glossopharyngeal nerve, cranial nerve IX. The greater horn and the lower part of the body of the hyoid bone are derived from this arch, as are the common and internal carotid arteries. The only muscle associated with the third arch is the stylopharyngeus muscle.

The arches four and six are both associated with the vagus nerve, cranial nerve X.

Pharyngeal arch four is associated with the superior laryngeal branch whilst arch six is associated with the inferior laryngeal branch.

From the fourth arch derive the muscles of the soft palate and all the skeletal muscles of the pharynx other than those from the third arch.

The thyroid, cricoid, arytenoid, cuneiform and corniculate cartilages are derived from this arch, as is the arch of the aorta and the proximal part of the subclavian artery.

The sixth arch is responsible for the ductus arteriosus and part of the right and left pulmonary arteries, all the muscles of the oesophagus and the intrinsic muscles of the larynx.

These later two arches together give rise to the larynx.

At the end of the fourth week of intrauterine life the floor of the pharynx consists of the five pharyngeal arches, (Larsen 4th edition.)

As the development of the tongue begins the ventral surface is attached to the floor of the mouth, as the foetus grows the attachment regresses in the anterior region and is then only attached posteriorly by what we know as the frenulum. If there is little or no regression then ankyloglossia or tongue-tie results.

The result of this embryological development is that the face is made up of fifteen different bones.

The bony face hangs from the inferior surface of the sphenoid and the frontal bones and is comprised of the ethmoid, two zygoma, two maxillae, two palatines, two nasal bones, two lacrimal bones, two inferior conchae and the vomer and the mandible.

The face contains the eyes, the sinuses, the oro and nasopharynx and the hypoglossal area including the tongue. I will visit these areas in more detail later.

I will deal with each bone of the face separately and the osteopathic techniques associated with them.

This will enable you to apply these techniques when dealing with clinical problems that are discussed later in this book. But only when you have evaluated and formulated your treatment plan.

The Sphenoid

The sphenoid sits in the centre of the cranial base. I see this bone as the orchestrator or conductor within the bony cranium because of its relationship with the bones associated with it and also the membrane.

The sphenoid articulates with the occiput, the parietals, the temporal bones, the palatine bones, the ethmoid, the vomer and the zygomae.

I do not intend to go into detail regarding the osteology and the ossification as I feel this is dealt with very well in Magoun's book Osteopathy in the Cranial Field.

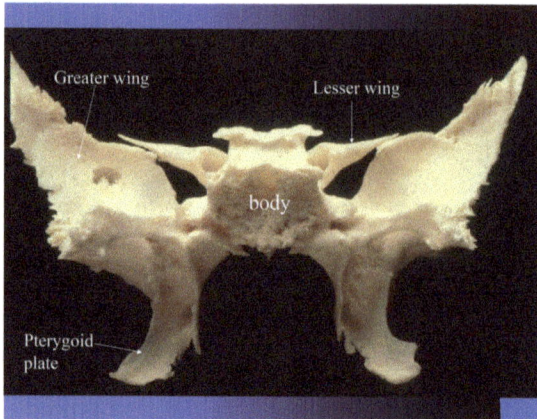

These slides of the sphenoid show how it has
a great influence on the rest of the cranium.

The sphenoid and the occiput work in tandem forming the cranial
base. As the cranial base rises the involuntary mechanism (IVM)
as we know it goes into the flexion phase and the greater wings
rotate anteriorly and laterally, everything laterally rotates and
shortens superiorly and inferiorly. As the cranial base lowers the
IVM goes into the extension phase, everything internally rotates
and the body becomes longer and thinner.

The sphenoid is a complicated bone with some very powerful
articulations. To release any restrictions associated with the
sphenoid I find it easier to first balance the membrane around the
sphenoid and the sella turcica. Once this is achieved you can use
quite simple techniques to disengage the greater wing from the
frontal, temporal bone and the zygoma.

With the patient supine, place two fingers on the frontal bone
adjacent to the articulation with the greater wing of the sphenoid.
Palpate the greater wing by sliding the fingers of your other hand
along the superior border of the zygomatic arch; the greater wing
is just medial to this and you can put your finger on it. Now
engage the mechanism, palpating the flexion and extension phases
of movement. When you are comfortable with this, the next time

the mechanism goes into flexion you hold back on the frontal bone and disengage the articulation between it and the sphenoid.

The same can be done with the temporal bone by using a five finger hold of the temporal bone (which is described in detail later) and with the same hold on the sphenoid you can disengage these two bones again in the flexion phase.

Similarly, if you need to release the sphenoid zygoma articulation you again palpate the greater wing of the sphenoid and you can either take a two finger hold on the zygoma externally or slide your first finger along the upper teeth until you reach the sulcus of the underside of the zygoma. You can now lift the zygoma away from the greater wing in the flexion phase of movement.

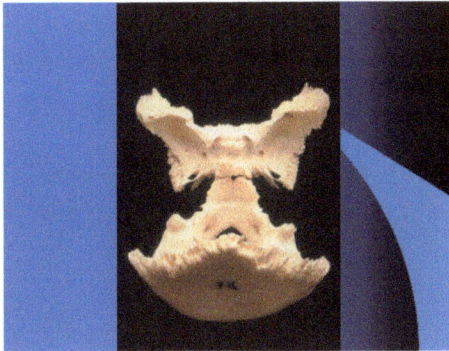

The sphenoid/occiput articulation. Note the serrated articulations for the frontal, temporal and parietal bones. Used with permission of the Willard/Carreiro Collection

The sphenoid is the key to all movement in the face and the cranium as it moves it takes all the bones associated with it in the same direction.

The Temporal Bone

Although not truly part of the face, the temporal bone has a great effect on everything around it. The muscles attached to it have a great influence in what happens to the face.

The temporal bone is comprised of three parts, the squamous (scale like), the mastoid (breast like) and the petrous (rock like). It is situated in the middle of the base of the skull, and in my mind conveys movement from the posterior aspect of the skull to the anterior aspect and vice versa.

It articulates with the occiput, the parietals, the sphenoid, the zygomae and the mandible.

It also can affect every cranial nerve from cranial nerve 3 to cranial nerve 11. The internal carotid artery passes through the carotid canal and therefore can be compromised in lesions of the temporal bone. Cranial nerve 6, the abducens, passes under the petro-sphenoid ligament, which passes from the tip of the petrous temporal to the sphenoid. In passing under this ligament, the nerve can be compromised if there is a lesion of the temporal bone and is a possible cause of strabismus in a child due to the effect on the lateral rectus muscle.

The cervical musculature and fascia have a great effect on the working of the temporal bone via the attachment to the occiput, which in turn can be influenced by the facia and musculature of the dorsal spine. Hence when we are treating the temporal bone, we have to look at the whole body.

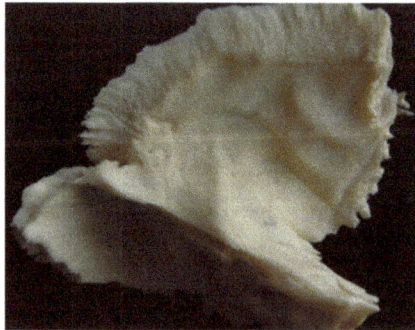

The petrous and squamous parts of the temporal bone.

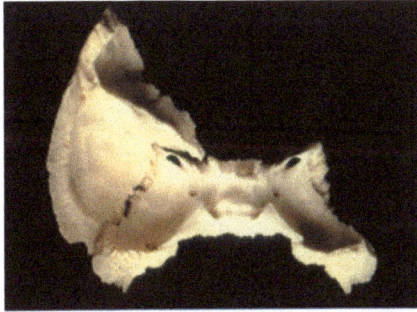

Inferior aspect of the temporal bone and
articulation with the sphenoid.
Used with permission of the Willard/Carreiro Collection

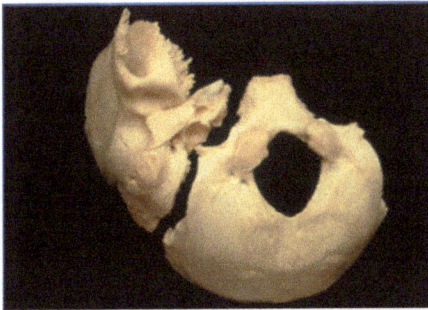

Inferior aspect of the temporal bone showing the mastoid and
the articulation with the occiput.
Used with permission of the Willard/Carreiro Collection

The petrous part of the temporal bone has an articulation with the occiput along the inferior border, the jugular surface has an irregular articulation which is grooved allowing movement and the mastoid component has an articulation with the occiput at the occipital mastoid suture.

The squamous part of the temporal bone and the parietal bones have a wonderful gill-like articulation that allows the temporal bone to slide during its articulation with the parietal bone, which allows it to rotate internally and externally.

Before releasing the sphenotemporal articulation you must observe and pay attention to the coronal and sagittal suture. Once these are moving well, you can then release the parietal from the squamous temporal bone.

To release any restrictions of the parietal temporal articulation, have your patient supine and then place your thumb of one hand along the parietal bone just above the articulation with the temporal bone. With the other hand, have the thumb along the squamous temporal and the thenar eminence and the fifth and ring fingers along the mastoid part of the temporal bone. If you gently take the temporal bone into external rotation you can spring the parietal temporal articulation in such a way that you can find any restrictions within that articulation, then by finding a fulcrum you can disengage the parietal and temporal bones and restore good mobility.

The articulation with the sphenoid is primarily with the greater wing, and the petrous portion and these articulations are described very well in anatomy books.

The zygomatic articulation will be shown in detail when we look at the zygoma and the treatment of the auditory tube and the temporomandibular joint.

You can see by the illustrations that the temporal bone has a huge influence on the mobility and function of the cranial base and through that the face.

The infratemporal muscles play a large role in the workings of the naso/oropharynx.

We will see further on in this book how important this bone is and the techniques we employ to balance it.

However, there is one technique, a Sutherland technique, which I feel is appropriate here.

To balance the two temporal bones.

With the operator sitting at the head of the patient, have your hands under the head with the mastoid process of the temporal bone resting on your thumbs and thenar eminences. You now have both temporal bones in your hands.

Engage the mechanism and when you are comfortably feeling the flexion and extension phases you can take direct control. Take one temporal bone into internal rotation and the other into external rotation. It is like wringing out a cloth. You take the two temporal bones to the extremes of their movement. Think what is happening to the membrane running along the petrous ridge, it is being wound up. Eventually you will come to a point where there is no more movement. Wait, and you will gradually feel the two bones begin to unwind and become very wide. Continue "watching" with your hands as the mechanism takes up a new phase and you will be surprised how mobile and balanced the temporal bones are.

In the course of this book you will see that the temporal bone has a great effect on so many structures and conditions. Techniques involving the temporal bone are described in different chapters.

However, we cannot leave the temporal bone without considering the articulation with the occiput. As I said previously, this articulation is often compromised due to the effects of the cervical musculature.

To release this articulation, you rotate the temporal bone externally and with the other hand you take hold of the squamous portion of the occiput and take it inferiorly and posteriorly at the same time as rotating it to find a fulcrum or point of balance.

The other method is to use what is commonly known as a fluid drive or V spread technique.

With one hand have your hand under the occiput with the first and middle fingers either side of the occipital mastoid suture forming a V. The first and middle fingers of the other hand are placed at the opposite diagonal on the frontal bone. Your intention is then to create energy and fluid to release the occipital mastoid suture. It is as though you are pumping fluid through the head on a diagonal axis. Of course, this is not possible as the brain, although containing a lot of fluid, is quite solid.

What I feel you do is engage the cerebrospinal fluid surrounding the brain and use its energy and strength to focus on one spot which will free the articulation.

Sutherland called the temporal bone "the trouble maker" within the head. When restricted in its movement it can affect so many other structures. I cannot recall many times that when working with the mechanism I have not had to rectify lesions associated with the temporal bone.

The Frontal Bone

The face hangs off the frontal bone.

It is a vault bone and is formed in membrane. At birth it is two distinct bones divided by the metopic suture, which often does not fuse completely until the age of six, although in approximately ten per cent of adults it remains patent.

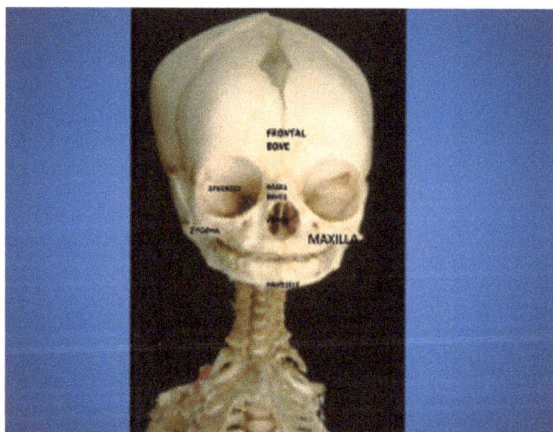

Infant skull.
Used with permission of the Willard/Carreiro Collection

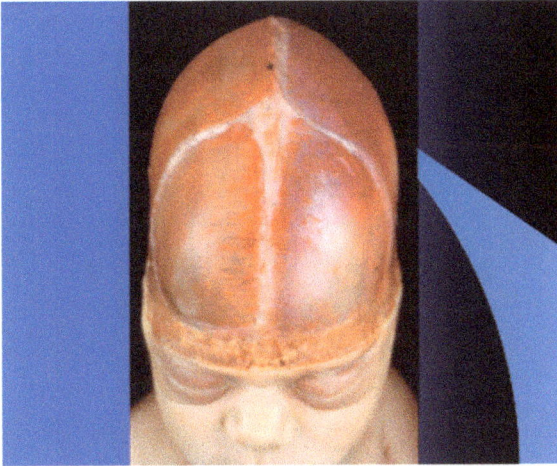

Frontal bone of term infant, note the metopic and coronal sutures.
Used with permission of the Willard/Carreiro Collection

As osteopaths we always consider the frontal bone as two separate components.

The frontal bone forms the superior aspect of the face and the roof of the orbit of the eye.

It has articulations with the parietal bones, the ethmoid, the sphenoid, the zygoma, the nasal bones, the maxillae and the lacrimal bones.

The anterior nasal component in the medial aspect is where the nasal bones and the maxilla articulate. These articulations are heavy serrated articulations, which allow some movement as these paired structures external and internally rotate during the flexion and extension phases.

Laterally there is a large articulation with the greater wing of the sphenoid bone.

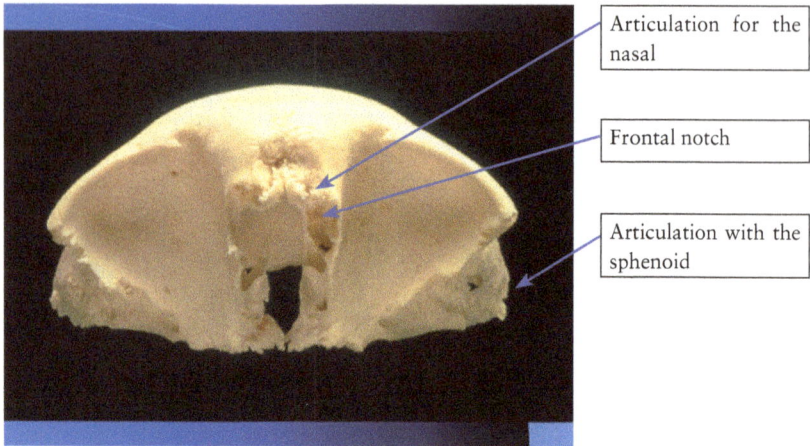

The frontal bone from anteroinferior angle. Note the articulations
for the nasal and maxilla bones and the ethmoid notch.
Used with permission of the Willard/Carreiro Collection

It is the sphenoid that moves the frontal bone during the flexion
and extension phase within the mechanism.

The frontal bone will move laterally, slightly forward and
inferiorly in flexion phase as the sphenobasilar junction rises and
medially and superiorly in the extension phase as the sphenobasilar
junction lowers. This movement has the effect of widening and
narrowing the ethmoidal notch as the glabella recedes.

Movement is transmitted to the frontal bone via the gearing
articulations between the two bones. Closer observation of the
articulations will reveal a tightly packed serrated articulation
between the lesser wing of the sphenoid and the frontal adjacent
to the frontal notch and a much heavier serrated articulation
between the greater wing and the anterolateral aspect of the
frontal bone. These serrations are wider and very pronounced,
which allows for the greater movement between the greater wing
of the sphenoid and the lateral aspect of the frontal bone.

Immediately anterior and inferior to the sphenoid articulation is the articulation with the zygoma. It is a serrated articulation that allows the zygoma to swivel slightly as it moves.

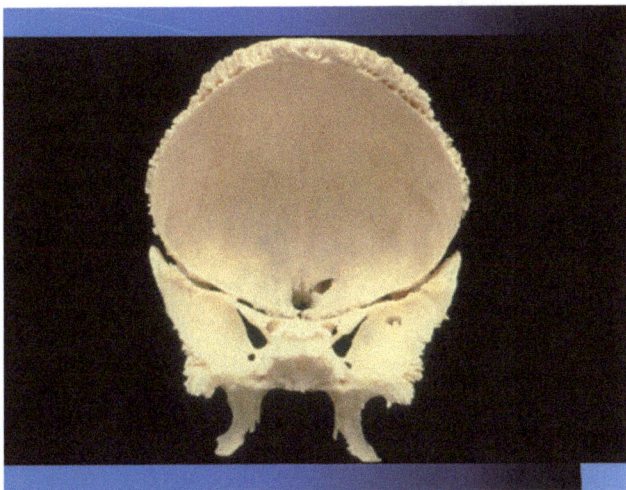

Note the articulation of the lesser wing of the sphenoid
with the posterior aspect of the frontal bone. Also note
the large gearing articulation of the greater wing.
Used with permission of the Willard/Carreiro Collection

The frontal bone forms the roof of the orbit of the eye. You will notice that there is a difference between the orbital ridge of a male and that of a female. The ridge is thicker in males than females.

Often when treating children and adults it is necessary to lift the frontal bone away from the bone's posterior to it. This will improve its mobility and at same time widen the ethmoid notch which will allow more freedom and improved mobility to the ethmoid bone and its attachments. Also think what is happening to the membrane as you lift the frontal bone, how this procedure affects the membrane as it is attached to the crista galli therefore affecting the sinuses especially the sagittal sinus where the cerebrospinal fluid (CSF) is being reabsorbed through the arachnoid granulations.

There are number of ways to lift the frontal bone.

The first one is to have the fingers of both hands on the frontal bone in the sagittal plane. The fingers rest just above the superior part of the orbit.

The frontal bone has to be lifted in the extension phase as the mechanism is becoming long and thin. In the flexion phase the frontal is going caudally and spreading laterally.

As the mechanism goes into the extension phase you lift the frontal away from the sphenoid and parietals.

You have overridden the mechanism; this is a direct technique. The frontal will seem to rise up and up and then reach a point where it cannot go any further, as though it is on elastic, when it reaches the extreme of the movement, I find that it tends to wobble a little as it begins to resolve. Finally, it will reach a point of stillness and eventually it will begin to return. As it begins to return you can widen the frontal, thus opening the ethmoid notch further.

The above technique is fine but my favoured technique gives you more control and is extremely good to use in the treatment of babies and children.

Have your dominant hand, in my case the right hand, across the frontal with the hypothenar eminence resting on the lateral aspect and the ring finger and the fifth digit (the little finger) spread across the frontal bone. Your elbow is resting on the pillow next to the head which allows you to have a soft hand.

Your other hand is under the occiput so that you can be in contact with the membrane at the confluence of the tentorium and the falx cerebri. The same method is employed as before where you lift the frontal at approximately 45 degrees away from the sphenoid and parietals in the extension phase. Reach a point where there is no more movement, then stillness. Then allow the frontal to return, opening the hand to encourage the widening of the ethmoid notch.

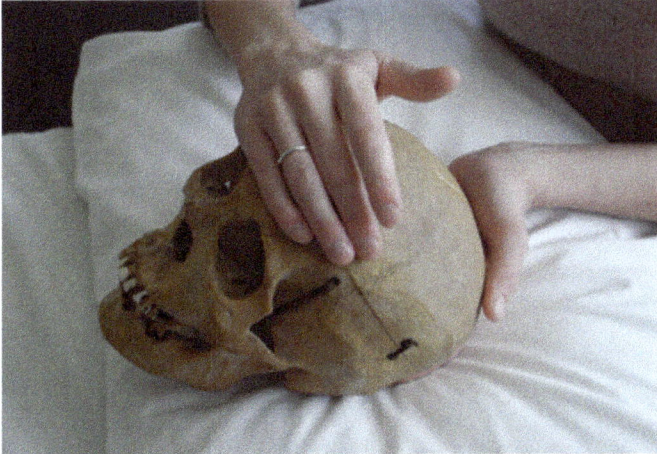

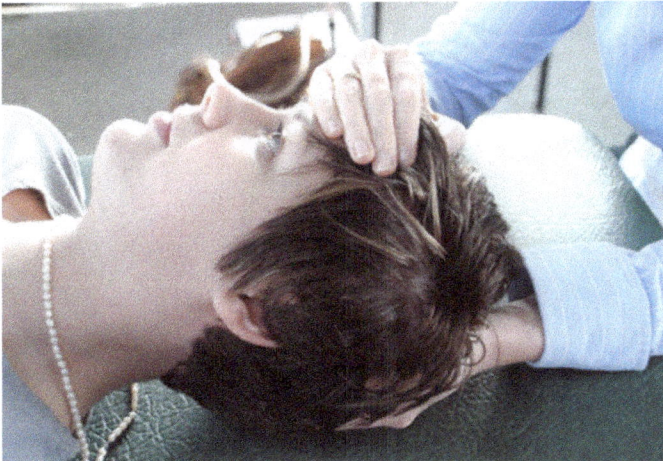

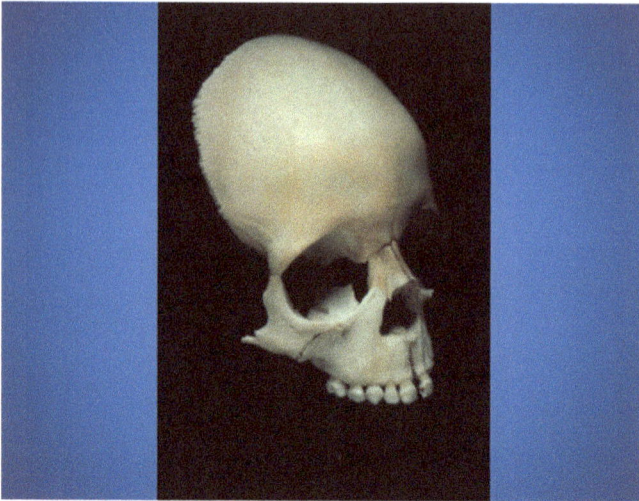

Let us now look at the bones associated with and articulate with the frontal bone and the sphenoid. To do this I will work from the midline of the face and move laterally.

The Nasal Bones

These two small bones hang off the anteromedial aspect of the frontal bone. The articulation between the two nasal bones is roughly the midline of the face. They form what is commonly known as the bridge of the nose.

The nasal bones articulate by a heavy serrated articulation that forms a very solid area and yet allows a certain degree of movement. These two bones form a protection for the articulation of the maxillae and the ethmoid bones which lie behind them.

The nasal bones are very solid structures and have a harmonic articulation with each other, the external surface is concavo-convex from above downwards and convex from side to side. They also articulate with the maxillae posteriorly and the nasal cartilage inferiorly. "The bones are ossified from one centre which appears at the beginning of the third month of intrauterine life in the membrane overlying the anterior part of the nasal capsule." (Gray's Anatomy)

As they are paired structures, they externally rotate in the flexion phase and internally rotate in the extension phase of their physiological motion.

Clinically, by understanding the movement of these components, it is possible to repair damage to the nasal cartilage, especially if seen soon after an accident. These are often patients who have been hit in the face playing a sport such as hockey or rugby or walked into something hard.

The technique is quite simple. With one hand gently engage the nasal bones between the thumb and either the first finger or the index finger. With the other hand take contact on the frontal bone over glabella with the middle finger. As the mechanism goes onto the flexion phase hold the frontal bone back by taking it posteriorly towards the occiput. The nasal bones will be moving into flexion, so will be externally rotating, gently disengage and release the nasal bones from the frontal. Remember that they are paired structures and will begin to orientate themselves around their own fulcrum. Follow the movement of the nasal bones and balance them around their own axis on to the frontal bone.

In sports injuries where the cartilaginous part of the nose has been damaged and often pushed to one side or impacted you can adjust the cartilaginous attachment to the nasal bones.

With your first finger and thumb on one hand, contact and engage the nasal bones. With the other hand take contact with the nasal cartilage in the same manner, i.e. with the first finger and thumb. In the flexion phase gently disengage the cartilage from the nasal bones and let it find a balance point in the midline to allow the nasal bones and the cartilage to reengage.

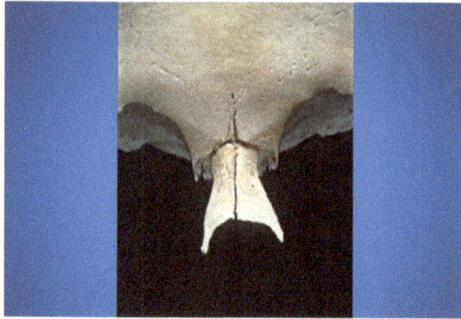

Nasal bones articulating with the frontal bone.

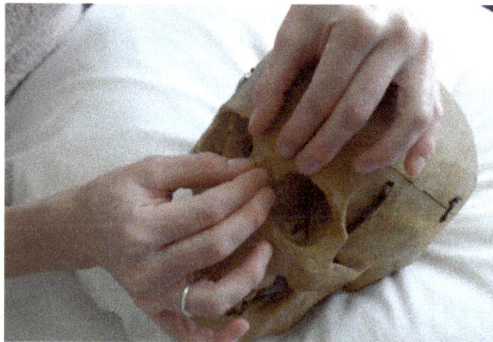

Disengagement of the nasal bones from the frontal bone.

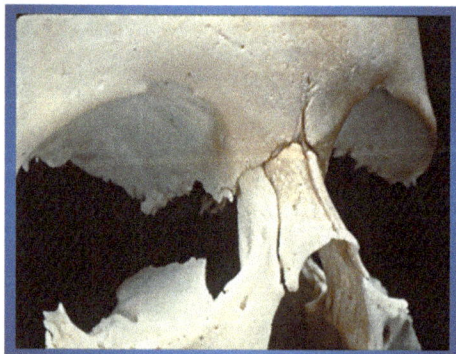

Nasal bones and maxilla in situ. Notice how they engage
deep into the frontal bone.
Used with permission of the Willard/Carreiro Collection

The Maxilla and Speed Reducers

The maxillae hang from the frontal bone and the articulation is directly posterior and lateral to the nasal bones. They are the largest bones in the face, they form the roof of the mouth, the floor and the lateral wall of the nasal cavity and they also form the floor of the orbit.

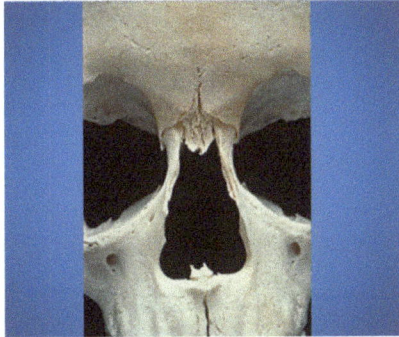

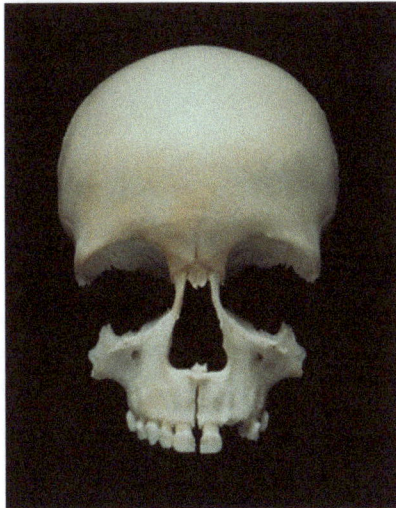

The articulation of the maxillae lies inferiorly
and laterally to the nasal bones.
Used with permission of the Willard/Carreiro Collection

The maxillae are pyramidal in shape. The anterior surface forms the cheek; the superior surface forms the floor of the orbit, medially is the nasal notch and inferiorly there is the housing for the upper teeth and the anterior aspect of the hard palate. Each maxilla also contains a large air sinus.

The maxillae hang from the frontal bone by a serrated articulation that allows movement to take place. They lay behind the nasal bones also articulate with them, they also articulate with the lacrimals, the ethmoid, palatines, vomer, zygomae, the inferior conchae and each other.

Movement of the maxillae is as follows. They are suspended from the frontal bone and as the sphenobasilar synchondrosis moves superiorly during the flexion phase, the posterior border moves posterolaterally thus widening the alveolar notch and the intermaxillary suture moves inferiorly and posteriorly.

The maxillae do not have any direct articulation with the sphenoid bone

The reason for this is that it is considered that the movement of the viscerocranium is too powerful to be directly transmitted to the middle face and the maxillae.

However, the sphenoid does move the maxilla indirectly by what osteopaths know as speed reducers.

This is a gearing mechanism that transfers movement from the sphenoid to the maxilla. Three bones directly articulate with the sphenoid and also the maxillae.

These bones are from medially to laterally, the vomer, the palatine and the zygoma. They move the maxillae through the midline, medial and lateral planes by their different forms of articulation and we will deal with them separately.

The first speed reducer is the vomer

The vomer is the midline speed reducer.

It is thin and flat and trapezoidal in shape. It is attached to the rostrum of the body of the sphenoid bone, by means of a thick elliptical border that surrounds the rostrum, like a pair of lips.

It articulates with the sphenoid, palatines, maxillae, ethmoid and the nasal septum.

Inferiorly it articulates with the maxillae anteriorly and the palatine bones posteriorly.

Its movement is like a ploughshare so that in flexion it drives the two bones inferiorly and laterally. By communicating with the maxilla directly and via the palatine bones posteriorly along its horizontal plate it is able to transfer movement from the sphenoid to the maxillae.

As the vomer moves in the flexion phase it moves the maxilla into external rotation with the posterior aspect going inferiorly, in this way it imparts the movement of the sphenoid to the maxilla.

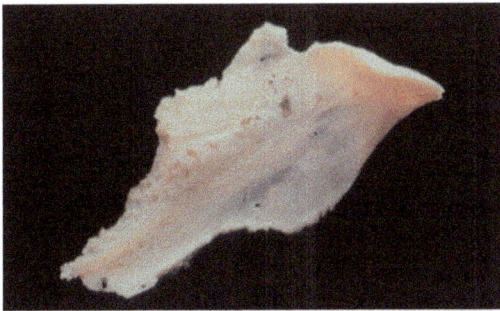

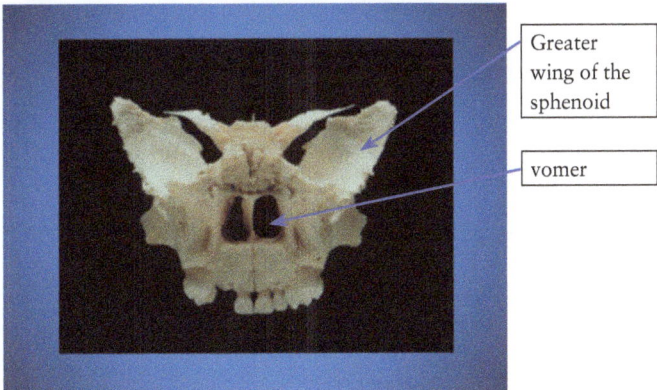

Greater wing of the sphenoid

vomer

Inferiorly the vomer runs from the palatine
bones to the anterior aspect of the mandible.
Used with permission of the Willard/Carreiro Collection

This osteopathic technique application to release the vomer and improve the movement often has a dramatic effect. Patients often comment that, after the vomer is released, they can breathe more easily, and it feels as though the whole of the area behind the nose has expanded and become free.

It is called the vomer pump technique

Standing beside your patient make sure that you are relaxed and your shoulders are loose and your hands soft.

Ask the patient to open their mouth and with a gloved hand insert your first finger along the midline to the crux where the maxillae and palatines meet.

Do not press upwards. This finger is a listening finger; it will palpate movement and the changes that occur.

With your other hand, place it across the frontals towards the sphenoid. It is often not possible to have your middle finger and thumb on the greater wings of the sphenoid especially if you have small hands. So as the frontal bone is doing exactly what the sphenoid is doing, if your hands are small or the patient has a large head contacting the frontal is sufficient.

The object of this technique is to follow the flexion and extension phases of the movement and when you are comfortable you override the mechanism. It is a direct technique and you take charge of the mechanism.

The next time the mechanism goes into the flexion phase follow the movement, you take the frontal/sphenoid deep into what I call "forced flexion" and keep it there. Do not allow the mechanism to come back into the extension phase.

With the finger in the mouth you are palpating and you wait, everything will become silent. You will not feel any movement.

It is as though the whole mechanism has become a deep black hole. When you find this point of total silence release the hand on the frontal/sphenoid and feel what is happening to the finger in the mouth.

You will feel the finger being drawn superiorly as the extension phase begins. It is very powerful and it often feels that this movement goes on for quite some time. Eventually the mechanism will begin another phase.

Now go back and take a vault hold and examine the mechanism. It will feel entirely different. More expressive, freer and the vomer can now articulate with the maxillae more positively. It can take the movement from the sphenoid to maxillae in the midline. At the same time, it will release the movement of the ethmoid and then nasal septum.

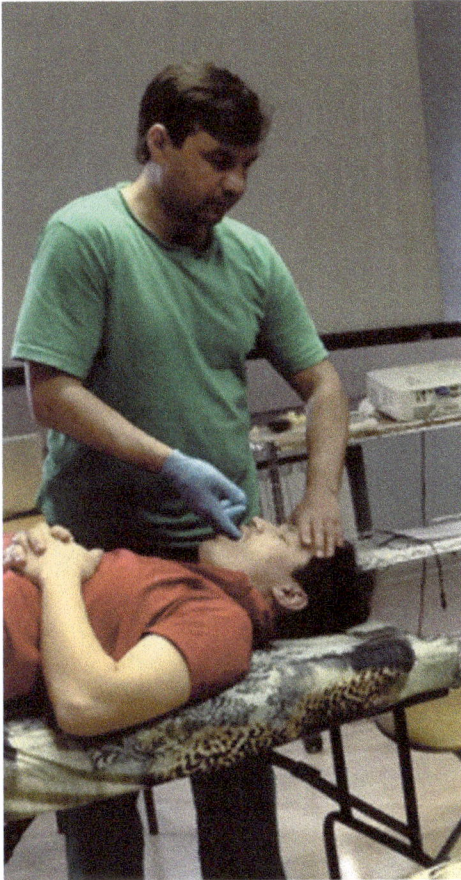

Vomer pump technique

49

The second speed reducer is the palatine bone

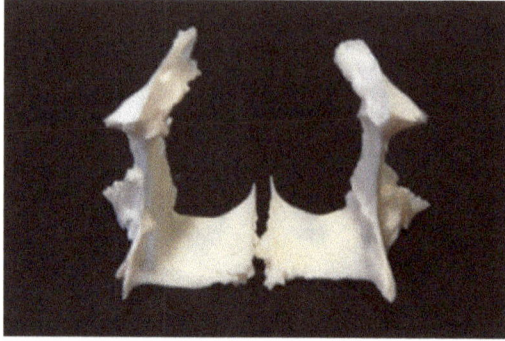

Palatine bones.

The palatine bones articulate with the maxillae, ethmoid, vomer, inferior conchae and the other palatine bone.

The bones fit posteriorly in the nasal cavity between the maxillae and the pterygoid processes of the sphenoid bone.

The sphenoid articulates directly with the palatine via the pterygoid plates. The pterygoid fits into two grooves in the posterior aspect of the inferior part of the perpendicular plate of the palatine. See below:

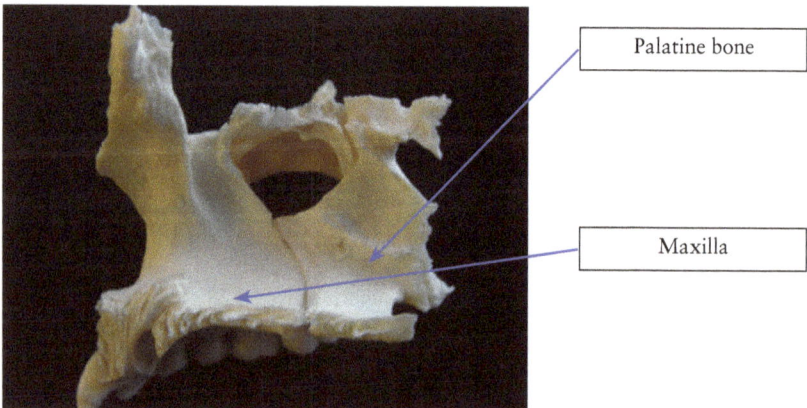

Lateral aspect of the palatine bone and the maxilla.

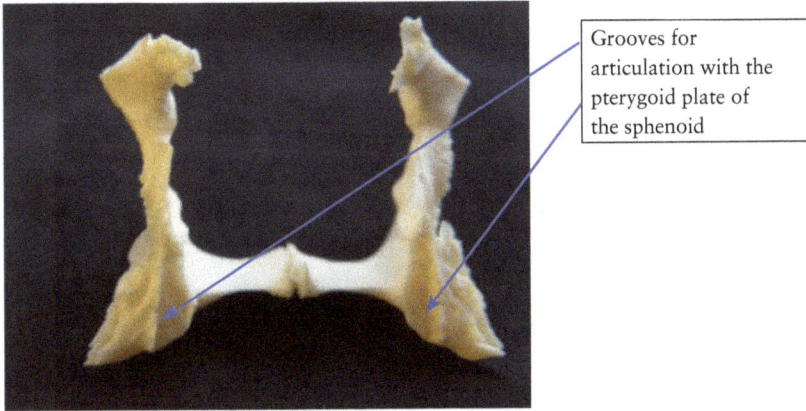

Grooves for articulation with the pterygoid plate of the sphenoid

Posterior aspect of the palatine bones.

In the flexion phase the pterygoid plates of the sphenoid bone take the palatine bone inferiorly and laterally and because of the palatines articulates with the maxilla, it takes the maxilla in the same direction.

The palatine is composed of a horizontal plate and a perpendicular plate.

The horizontal plate articulates with the other palatine and anteriorly with the maxilla. There is also a long vertical articulation with the maxilla in the lateral aspect.

On the superior aspect of the perpendicular plate is a small triangle of bone which forms part of the floor of the orbital cavity sitting between the orbital aspect of the ethmoid bone and the maxilla, which also forms part of the floor of the orbital cavity. The movement of the palatine bone is critical in the drainage of the fluid within the orbital cavity. The movement of the bones forming the orbital cavity allow a change of pressure and therefore a pumping movement to take place.

This triangle of bone on the superior aspect of the vertical plate of the palatine is clinically significant when you have young child with a blocked lacrimal duct.

The lacrimal gland is situated in the fossa of the frontal bone above the orbit of the eye. The duct transverses medially then inferiorly to finally ends at the naso/lacrimal duct on the lateral side of the nose. If the palatine bone is not moving comfortably with its articulation with the pterygoid plates the movement is compromised and good drainage does not take place.

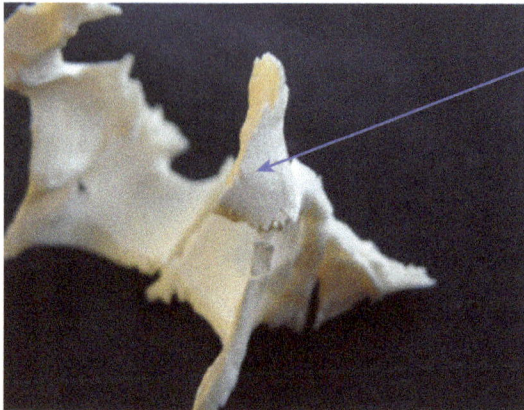

Orbital part of the palatine bone

Triangular area of the superior aspect of the palatine bone.

When the lacrimal duct becomes blocked, the baby tends to have crusting of the eyelids due to mucus building up on the surface of the eye and then drying. Although parents are often told that it will improve as the baby grows or they are sometimes offered surgery.

As osteopaths we can improve the mobility of the orbit, because the drainage is often compromised by the palatine bone not articulating properly with the ethmoid and maxilla and therefore not allowing a pumping action to take place.

It takes a great deal of practice in palpation to succeed in being able to solve the problems of the palatine bones.

You have to understand the anatomy and the applied anatomy of how this bone works. Remember it has a long articulation with the maxilla in the perpendicular plane laterally, as well as the attachment with the maxilla anteriorly.

However, the main problem is often found with the articulation with the pterygoid plates of the sphenoid.

If the pterygoid plates do not fit properly into the grooves in the posterior aspect of the palatine bone, the articulation between it and the pterygoid plates of the sphenoid do not move effectively therefore it does not allow the sphenoid to move the palatine in an inferior and lateral motion which follows the movement of the sphenoid in the flexion phase.

To release the palatine bone from grooves on the pterygoid plate is as follows (for a right-handed person):

With your patient either lying or sitting place your left hand across the sphenoid with your middle finger and your thumb on the greater wing. However, in most adults this is not possible to span the head coronally in such a way, especially if you have small hands. So, as before place your hand across the sphenofrontal articulation (whatever the movement of the sphenoid the frontal will do the same.) Now engage the mechanism in the flexion phase and the extension phases.

With your right hand, place the index or first finger in the mouth by sliding it along the medial border of the upper teeth of the maxilla until you reach the last molar. The palatine is directly posterior to the maxilla.

To engage the palatine bone, you have to move your finger posteriorly.

However, you do not wish to do this until you are ready to release the palatine from the pterygoid plates of the sphenoid bone.

With your left-hand monitoring flexion and extension, you override the mechanism by taking the sphenoid to the extreme of flexion, forcing it down thus making the pterygoid plates go as wide as possible. As you reach the extreme of flexion you simultaneously move your hand in the mouth posteriorly to the palatine bone past the molars, if you go too far the patient will gag, and forcibly push your finger laterally and palmar rotate the hand. This all happens in one motion. It is what I call an "in and out" technique, as soon as forced flexion is found, you palmar rotate the hand and take your finger out of the mouth.

This should allow the palatine to reseat in the grooves of the pterygoid plate.

The third speed reducer is the zygoma

The zygoma articulates with the frontal, sphenoid, temporal and maxilla. In my opinion it has a number of roles.

Because of the density of the bone, it acts to protect the eye both in the new born and the adult, it also transfers movement from the front of the face posteriorly and vice-versa.

It is a dense bone, shaped like a sail and it has a broad squamous articulation with the parietal bone and two articulations anteriorly, one with the frontal and the other larger one with the sphenoid. However, it is the articulation with the temporal bone that mainly allows transfer of movement to the maxilla.

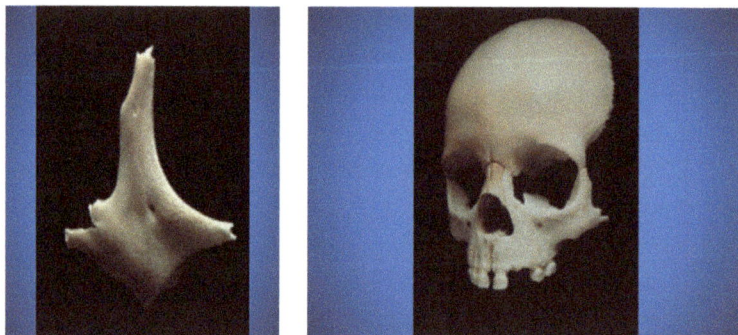

The zygoma articulating with the frontal and maxilla note the shape of the zygoma in the picture on the left.

The articulation with the temporal bone is very interesting, it is in the anterior third of the zygomatic arch and is a wonderful piece of anatomical engineering.

The inferior aspect of the temporal articulation with the zygoma is extremely smooth and is long.

The anterior articulation between the zygoma and the temporal bone is horizontal with two slits allowing the zygoma to fit into the temporal portion of the zygomatic arch. It allows the bones to rotate externally as the sphenoid takes the temporal bone into flexion and the two long smooth surfaces inferiorly and superiorly allowing the zygoma to slide externally in its movement. In this way the sphenoid, along with the frontal, transfers its movement to the maxillae.

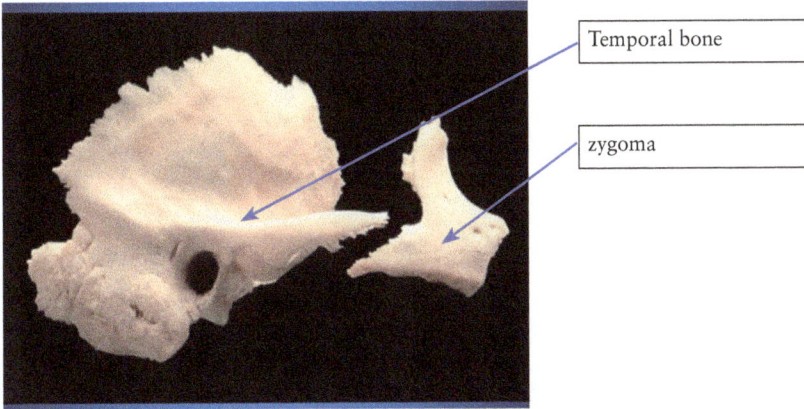

Temporal bone

zygoma

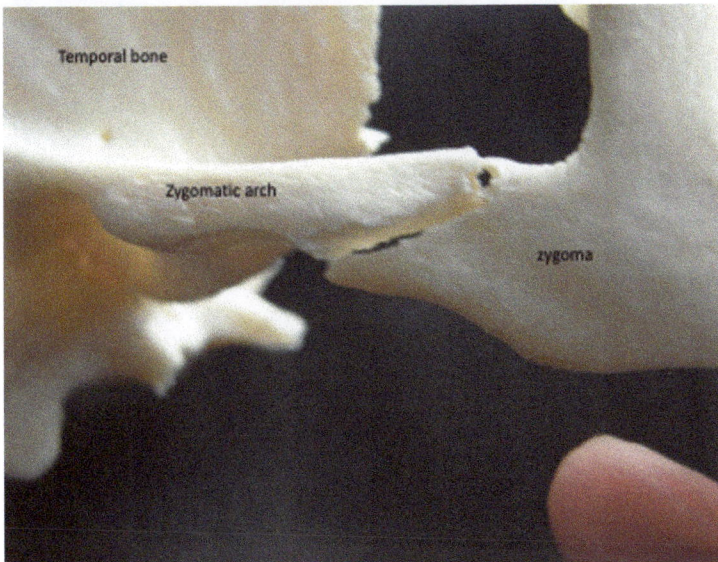

Temporal/zygoma articulation. Note the angle of the articulation.

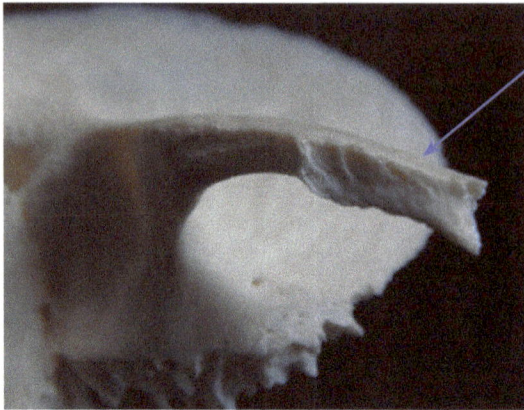

Inferior aspect of the articulatory surface of the temporal bone that articulates with the zygoma

Inferior smooth surface of the temporal part of the zygomatic arch.

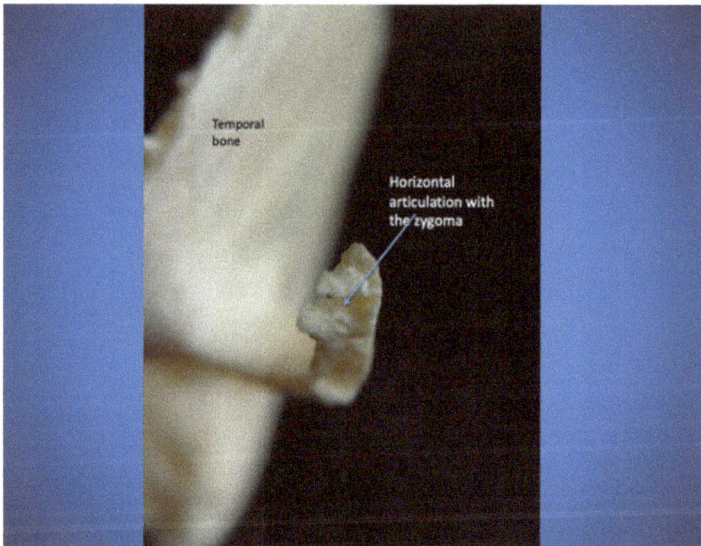

Temporal bone

Horizontal articulation with the zygoma

Note the two horizontal grooves of the temporal articulation.

I tend to use two techniques for releasing the zygoma.

The first is a simple disengagement, however the positioning of the fingers is extremely important. The objective is to release the articulation along the zygomatic arch.

Firstly, with one hand take a five finger hold of the temporal bone.

A five-finger hold is as follows.

Place your middle finger in the ear and with your first finger and thumb take a firm grip of the temporal portion of the zygomatic arch posterior to its attachment to the zygoma. This is very important as I find a lot of students place their fingers either too wide apart, therefore not taking a firm hold of the temporal arch or they are too far forward and either on the joint itself or on the zygoma. The ring finger rests on the mastoid process and the little finger (digit 5) on the occipital mastoid suture. You now have the whole of the temporal bone in your hand.

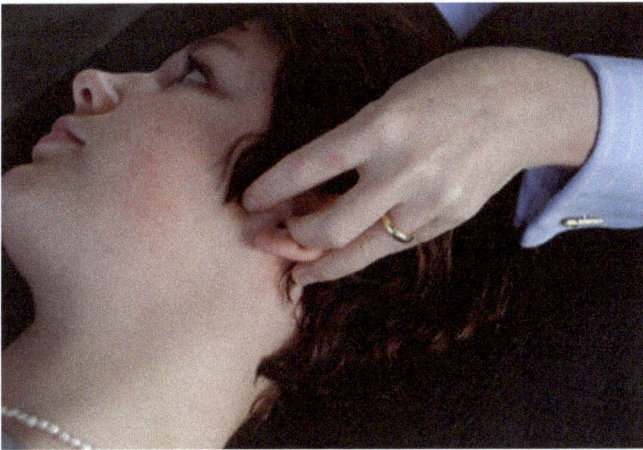

Five finger hold, note the middle finger in the ear
and the ring finger on the mastoid process.

With your other hand take a firm hold of the zygomatic part of the arch. Then engage the mechanism when you are comfortable, the next time the mechanism goes into flexion disengage the zygoma from the temporal bone, when it reaches the full extent of its movement let it come back it the extension phase. This is a direct technique, you override the mechanism.

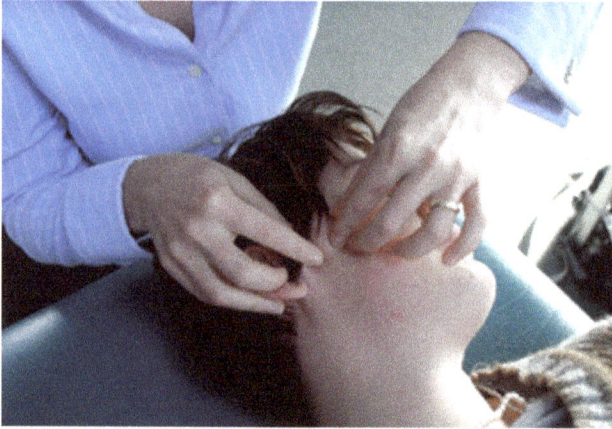

A firm grip is taken on the zygomatic part of the zygomatic arch.

The second technique is my preferred technique.

Stand on the opposite side to which you want to work. Have relaxed shoulders and soft hands.

Take the same five finger hold of the temporal bone, then with the other hand lift the gum with your first finger resting on the upper teeth. Fold the rest of your fingers into the palm of your hand keeping them away from the rest of the face and nose. Now slide your first finger along the upper teeth and go slightly cranially and you will find a sulcus which is the underside of the zygoma. If you go too far your finger will hit the mandible of the temporomandibular joint.

When you reach this sulcus slightly palmar rotate your hand so that the zygoma sits on your finger. Palpate the mechanism, feel flexion and extension, when the flexion phase occurs gently take the temporal bone into external rotation and at the same time ease the zygoma away from its articulation with the temporal bone along the zygomatic arch. Wait until you feel it reaches a point of balance. Remember this is a direct technique so you have overridden the mechanism. When you reach your point of balance or fulcrum, you should feel what I always think of as a little "sigh"; everything relaxes and you can come off and let the mechanism take over.

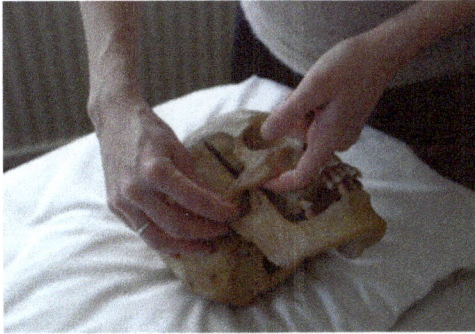

Operator standing, five finger hold with right hand and
first finger of the left hand under the zygoma in the sulcus.

You can use this technique for the articulations with the frontal,
sphenoid and maxilla moving your temporal hand to the
appropriate bone.

We have now seen how movement from the sphenoid bone to the
maxilla is transferred via interaction with the speed reducers. So,
the maxilla moves inferiorly and laterally in the flexion phase
along with the sphenoid.

The Ethmoid Bone

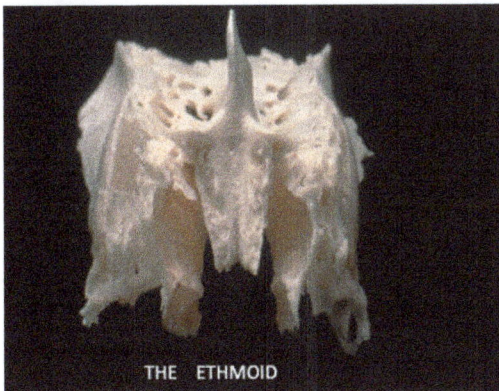

THE ETHMOID

Immediately posterior to nasal and maxillae bones is the ethmoid
notch of the frontal bone and within the notch sits the ethmoid bone.

59

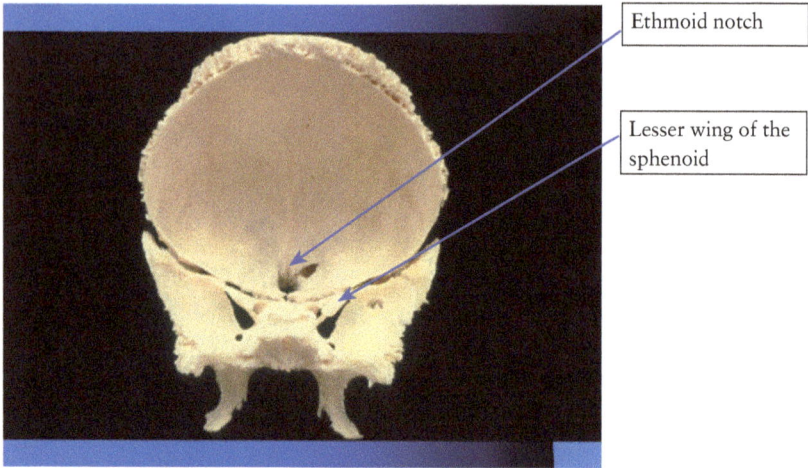

Sphenoid and frontal showing the lesser wing and
the ethmoid notch in the frontal bone.
Used with permission of the Willard/Carreiro Collection

The notch is horizontal and the lateral articulatory aspect is a smooth harmonic suture allowing mobility.

The sphenoid articulates with the ethmoid by means of a gomphosis where a protrusion from the midline of the sphenoid fits into a groove on the superior surface of the ethmoid posteriorly. This articulation allows the ethmoid bone to be moved by the sphenoid. In the flexion phase the sphenoid tips forward and in so doing the ethmoid is tipped inferiorly which in turn pushes the vomer, which is attached to the inferior surface of the ethmoid posteriorly in the opposite direction to the sphenoid.

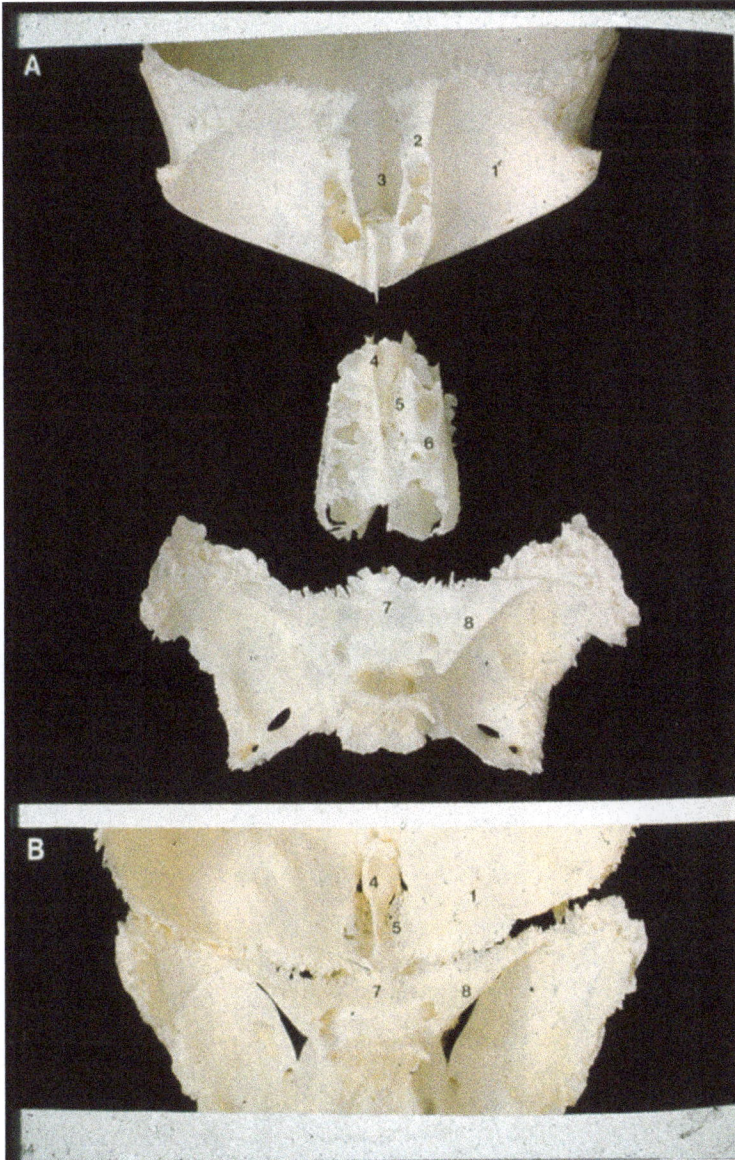

The ethmoid bone is complex. It has a midline plate and two lateral masses, which like all paired structures externally rotate in flexion and internally rotate in extension.

The body of the ethmoid bone is made up of numerous air cells which begin to develop in utero at about three months and are clinically relevant from the first year of life. They grow slowly and reach adult size by the age of twelve years.

The ethmoid bone has immense lightness and with a perpendicular plate and a horizontal cribriform plate which fills the ethmoid notch of the frontal bone and forms a large part of the roof of the nasal roof and is penetrated by many foramina which allow parts of the olfactory nerve to pass through.

The crista galli protrudes superiorly from the cribriform plate, with the falx cerebri attached to the crista galli. So as the membrane and especially the falx cerebri move within the motion of the involuntary mechanism, the falx pulls on the crista galli lifting it out of the ethmoid notch in the extension phase.

There are two lateral masses which sit like saddle bags either side of the perpendicular plate. During the flexion phase of involuntary motion, the perpendicular plate moves anteriorly and inferiorly and the lateral masses externally rotate.

The lateral walls of the ethmoid bone are very thin and as it can present clinically within the first year of life, cross infection can take place with the eye, which it is adjacent to, giving rise to orbital cellulitis.

The ethmoid bone is very delicate and has to be treated with great respect. When palpating, alight very gently onto the nasal bones which sit directly above the ethmoid.

Your touch should be as light as a butterfly alighting on a leaf.

Have one hand, say the left hand, under the occiput with the thumb along the sagittal sinus and falx cerebri while the right hand has the middle and ring fingers resting on the nose and the thumb resting on the forehead, then the first finger can gently alight onto the nasal bone and you can then palpate in depth to the ethmoid bone which is directly behind the nasal bones.

Also, by contacting the membrane and especially the falx with the thumb of your lower hand, you can engage the mechanism and as Sutherland said "ring the ethmoid bell" by taking the membrane and falx cerebri posteriorly. Thereby lifting the ethmoid out of the ethmoid notch via the falx cerebri and balancing the ethmoid in the midline via the perpendicular plate and the crista galli.

For its size the ethmoid has a considerable influence over the mechanism and if it is treated harshly can have disastrous effects, causing nausea and problems arising from the imbalance of the membrane.

When I was teaching many years ago on a postgraduate cranial course, I had the misfortune to be a victim of heavy-handed treatment of the ethmoid bone.

On this course there were a number of dentists from all over Europe. As we had odd numbers, I volunteered to be a model for a German dentist. The class was being guided through palpation of the ethmoid bone, its relationships and its movement by a very experienced osteopath.

As soon as the person put his hands on me, I realised how heavy-handed he was, pressing down firmly and hard on the nasal bones. I began to feel unwell and that my diaphragms were collapsing and I thought I was going to void my bladder. Suddenly he stopped as his hands were taken away by a colleague who saw me going very pale and struggling to breathe.

Two colleagues tried to repair the damage that had been inflicted as they thought the tentorium had gone into spasm somehow, I recovered but later in the day I fainted, which was very unlike me and for weeks following, I felt unwell.

The consequences of this very heavy-handed treatment were, that for the next three months I could not work with the involuntary mechanism and I had to be treated twice a week. For years after this incident I could not look up to the left without getting a sharp pain over my right eye.

The simple moral of this is that when working with the mechanism be gentle and respectful and only use as much force as is necessary.

This little bone can cause great problems if not treated with respect.

CHAPTER 5

The Auditory Tube/Eustachian Tube

To be successful in treating otitis media you have to understand the applied anatomy and the clinical pathology of the auditory tube.

In the adult the tube is about 36cm long, the bony aspect 12cm long and the cartilaginous part 24cm long.

When the baby is born the tube runs horizontally from the inferior border of the temporal bone anteriorly to the oro/nasopharynx. As the child grows and the shape of the cranial base changes and the angle increases. The angle of the tube in the sagittal plane increases to about 45 degrees by the age of six years and in the horizontal plane it increases to 30 degrees.

In some cases, as in Gray's Anatomy, the tube is known as the pharyngotympanic tube.

It connects the tympanic cavity to the nasopharynx and allows the passage of air between these spaces.

The auditory tube is a sinus and one of its functions is to evacuate detritus from the middle ear by letting it flow down the tube to the nasopharynx.

The auditory tube arises from the bony part of the inferior aspect of the temporal bone in the medial third.

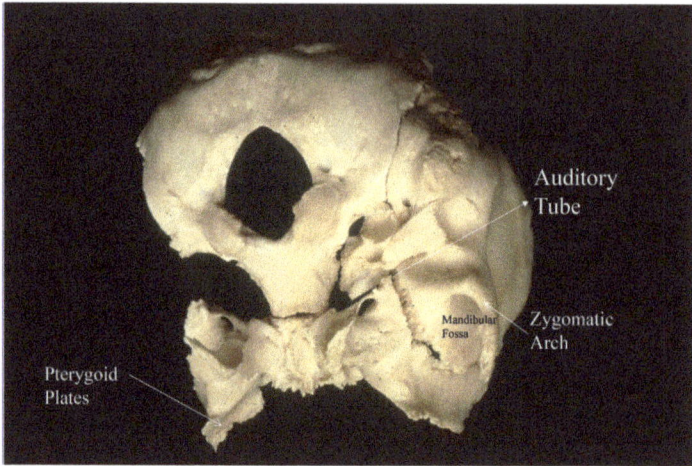

Used with permission of the Willard/Carreiro Collection

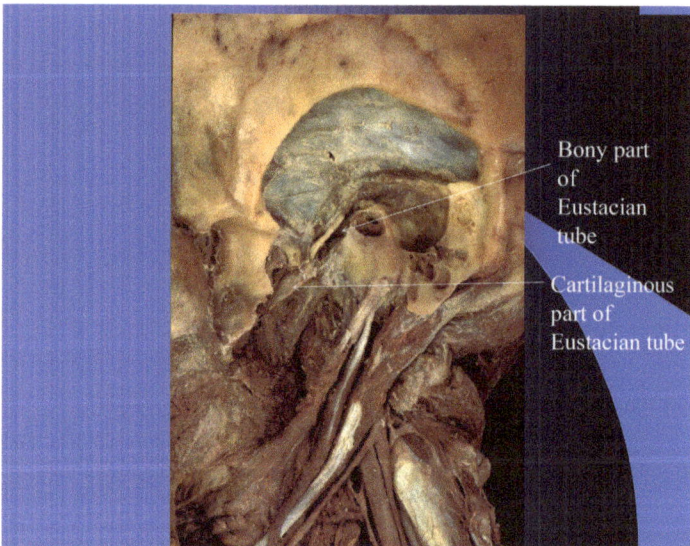

It then descends anteromedially and inferiorly as shown here.
Used with permission of the Willard/Carreiro Collection

The cartilaginous part of the tube eventually reaches the oropharynx at the palatine aponeurosis. This is formed from the tensor veli palatini muscle which, arising from the inferior border of spine of the sphenoid bone it descends with the tube and then continues laterally around the pterygoid hamulus to meet the tensor veli palatini muscle from the other side to form the palatine aponeurosis.

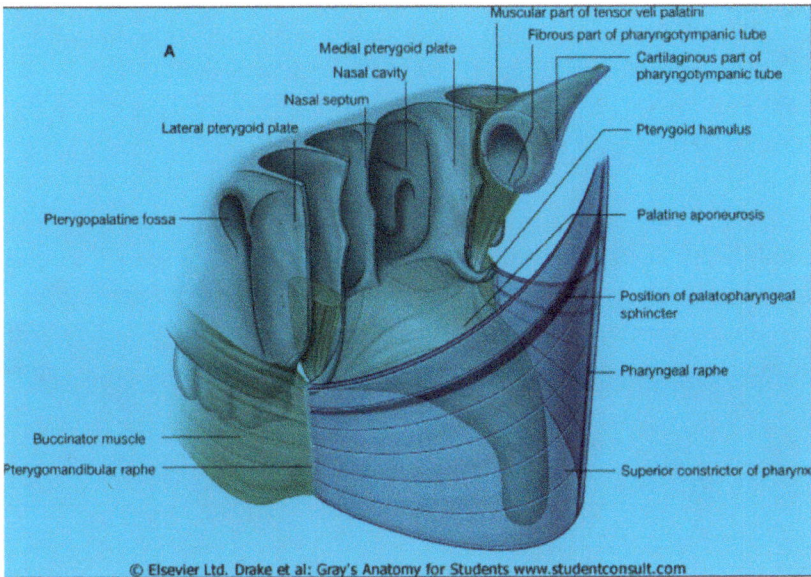

A — Medial pterygoid plate — Nasal cavity — Nasal septum — Lateral pterygoid plate — Pterygopalatine fossa — Buccinator muscle — Pterygomandibular raphe — Muscular part of tensor veli palatini — Fibrous part of pharyngotympanic tube — Cartilaginous part of pharyngotympanic tube — Pterygoid hamulus — Palatine aponeurosis — Position of palatopharyngeal sphincter — Pharyngeal raphe — Superior constrictor of pharynx

© Elsevier Ltd. Drake et al: Gray's Anatomy for Students www.studentconsult.com

To allow the oropharynx to function positively you have to be able to swallow and therefore change pressure within the oral cavity allowing a pumping action to take place. This pumping action allows a change of pressure within the oropharynx and the tube itself.

The palatine aponeurosis plays a large part in enabling that pressure change.

Imagine the tube as a tunnel divided horizontally so there is an upper and lower portion.

In an ideal world air proceeds up the roof or superior part of the tube from the oropharynx to the middle ear. Here the pressure of the air should move the detritus inferiorly along the lower part of the tube assisted by cilia in the lower part of the tube as it reaches the palatine aponeurosis. These cilia all beat in the same direction at the same time.

This mucocilary transport system is innervated by the parasympathetic nervous system via the sphenopalatine ganglion and the vidian nerve which is a branch of the trigeminal nerve.

The sympathetic supply is from the hypothalamus via the ganglion to the carotids. There is also self-regulation from the sensory cells within the mucosa.

The tube itself is protected by Ostmann's fatty tissue, which is a small layer of fatty tissue on the lateral side that closes across the tube, therefore preventing reflux entering the tube and getting into the middle ear. Mucosal associated lymphoid tissue (MALT) and goblet cells, mucin-secreting glands, also protect the tube from infection.

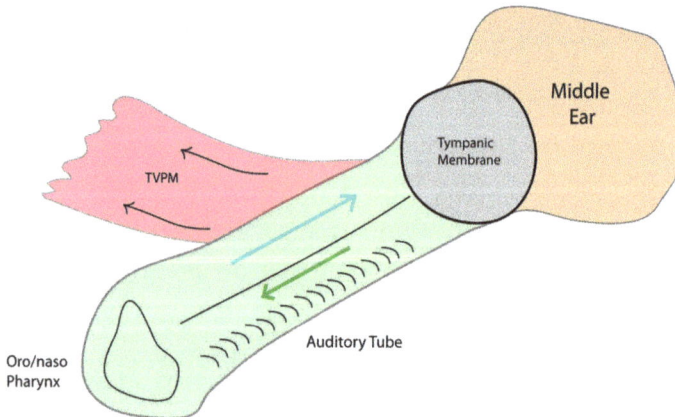

A diagram showing the auditory tube and
the adjacent component parts.

OSTEOPATHY WITHOUT BORDERS

As in the diagram above, you see the tensor veli palatini muscle attached to the lateral lamina. As the muscle contracts, it lifts the superior portion of the tube allowing aeration to take place. As the tensor veli palatini muscle relaxes, the elastin within the wall of the tube allows it to collapse thus producing a pumping action that will move air and detritus down the tube to oropharynx.

Below is a picture of a dissection of a baby. I have highlighted the two palatini muscles and the auditory tube is in blue.

You will see how these two muscles are associated with the tube as they descend to the oropharynx.

You will also note the middle ear and the mandibular division of the trigeminal nerve cranial nerve V as it passes through the foramen ovale and descends towards the mandible.

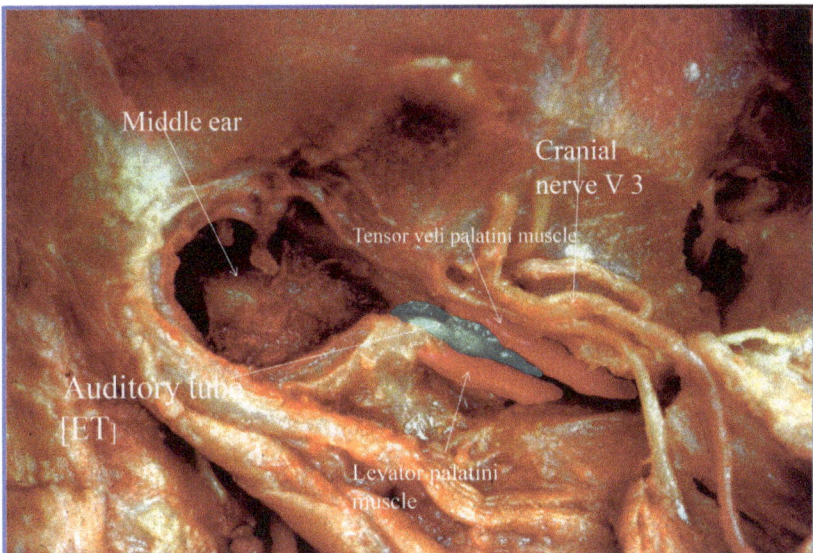

Used with permission of the Willard/Carreiro Collection

Otitis Media

One of the fascinating osteopathic challenges is treating children with otitis media, either acute or chronic.

I suppose that it is not surprising that the UK is the only country in the world to call chronic otitis media "glue ear". We Brits have an ingenious/unique way of describing things! Whatever name we give the condition however the effect is the same. The three small bones, the ossicles, the malleus, incus and stapes are not able to convey sound from the tympanic membrane to the oval window and thus to the cochlea due to a build-up of detritus within the middle ear.

Acute otitis media can occur from a very early age and medical opinion is that otitis media does not occur after the age of six years. I have not found that to be the case in practice.

I have seen children as old as 13 years with chronic otitis media and some of them were profoundly deaf.

So why does otitis media occur?

Firstly, you can have changes within the tube itself, either obstruction, abnormal pathology or intrinsic inflammation secondary to infection. Extrinsic factors such as tumours or adenoidal enlargement are also a cause. Finally, you could have a functional collapse of the tube compliance.

Other factors can affect the viscosity of the fluid within the tube such as inflammation, cystic fibrosis, viruses, bacterial infection, anticholinergic medication such as atropine which blocks acetylcholine, and antihistamines.

It is so important to examine the oropharynx carefully and if there are enlarged tonsils then you should recommend that they are removed.

The most common infection of the middle ear is from streptococcus pneumonia. Others that can cause infection are chlamydia trachomatis and haemophilus influenzae.

As osteopaths we rarely see acute otitis media. However, if you do then it can be effectively treated using osteopathic techniques.

Acute otitis media presents with a fever and otalgia and hearing loss. There is an effusion from the tube for up to three months and two out of three children have at least one episode before the age of one year. At three years of age 80 per cent have at least one episode and 50 per cent have up to three episodes. These children have a greater risk of middle ear disease.

Recurrent or chronic otitis media is very common and is usually due to defective drainage of the auditory tube.

Males more than females are affected, as are the lower socioeconomic groups. One factor that has been shown is that bottle feeding, especially in the horizontal position, can increase the probability of infection (if you look into a baby's mouth that has been bottle fed you can often see a milky covering of the oropharynx.)

Passive smoking is another important factor.

As osteopaths we have to maintain the integrity of the oropharynx by making sure the bony structure and the muscular attachments function as near normally as possible.

The body is a remarkable machine, every part of our body interacts with every other part whether it will be in small or large way. It is often to the amazement of patients that something which happens in the lower extremity or the pelvic floor can affect what happens to the rest of the body including the movements within the skull and the face.

The mobility of the bones of the skull and their associated muscles are constantly being affected by what is happening within the rest of the body.

So, when we approach a problem with the auditory tube, we must first look at the whole body and then at those structures intimately associated with the head and neck.

Changes in tension and movement of the muscles attached to the occiput and parietals can and do have a great effect on the way the temporal bone works and how this affects the muscles attached to it that play a big role in how the nasopharynx works.

We also have to assess the way the speed reducers, the vomer, palatine and the zygoma are working as they convey movement from the sphenoid to the maxillae.

Good movement of the maxillae and the speed reducers is essential if the drainage of the tube is effective.

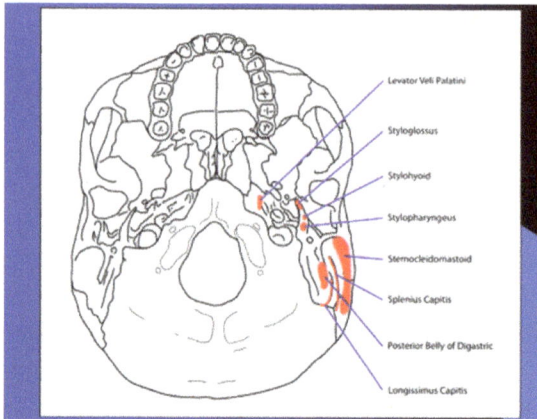

This is a diagram of the muscle attachments to the temporal bone; these muscles play important roles in maintaining the integrity of the oro/nasopharynx.

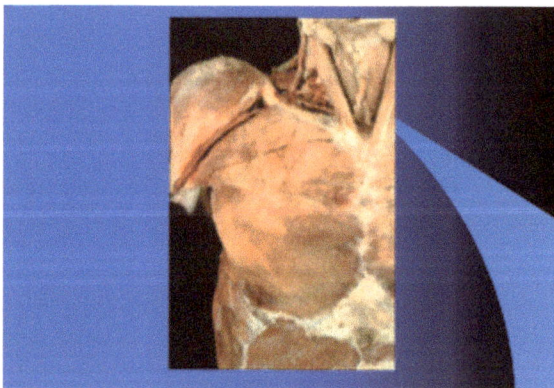

Sternocleidomastoid muscle showing the attachments
from the temporal bone to the clavicle and sternum.
Used with permission of the Willard/Carreiro Collection

Finally, once function has been restored, we have to make sure that the mediastinum has a freedom and a fluidity to it so that there is good drainage through the large vessels and the lymphatics.

The hyoid bone plays an important part in how the oropharynx works. It is the link between the muscles arising from the inferior aspect of the temporal bone and the soft palate.

It is often that the small things in anatomy can be have a large part in how the body works and this is the case with the little hyoid bone.

If you palpate the angle of your jaw and move your fingers medially you will come into contact with this amazing little bone that has such an effect on swallowing and the movement of the tongue.

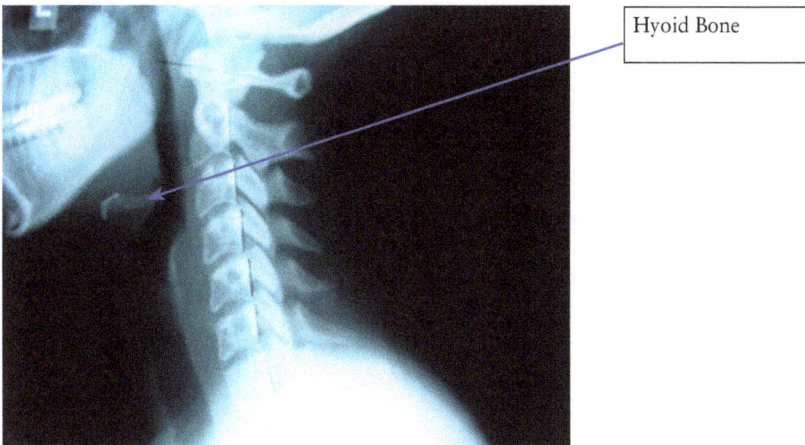

In this x-ray you can see the hyoid bone below
the mandible and anterior to the forth cervical vertebrae.

The hyoid swings freely and is not attached to any other bone, but has a number of important muscles either attached to it or associated with it.

The hyoid is comprised of a body and four lateral horns, two lesser and two greater. They are attached to the body by a secondary cartilaginous joint, thereby allowing some small movement.

Overall, ten muscles are attached to the hyoid bone as well as the fascial loop through which the digastric muscle passes on its way to the mandible.

They are: - The middle constrictor

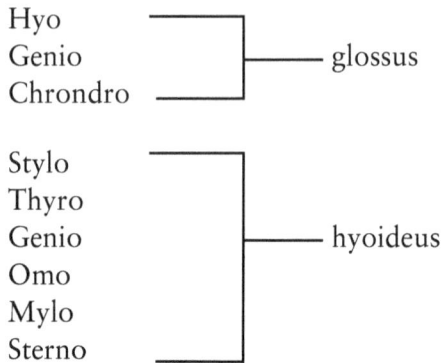

```
Hyo        ──────┐
Genio            ├──── glossus
Chrondro   ──────┘

Stylo      ──────┐
Thyro            │
Genio            ├──── hyoideus
Omo              │
Mylo             │
Sterno     ──────┘
```

The glossal muscles are attached to the greater horn and the hyoideal muscles either go superiorly to the mandible, the temporal bone or inferiorly to the scapula or the sternum thus stabilising the hyoid inferiorly.

Stylohyoid muscle descends from the styloid process of the temporal bone anteromedially to attach to the greater horn. However, on its descent it allows the digastric muscle arising from the digastric notch lateral to the styloid process on the inferior aspect of the temporal bone to pass through it on its pathway to the mandible where it acts as a depressor for the mandible.

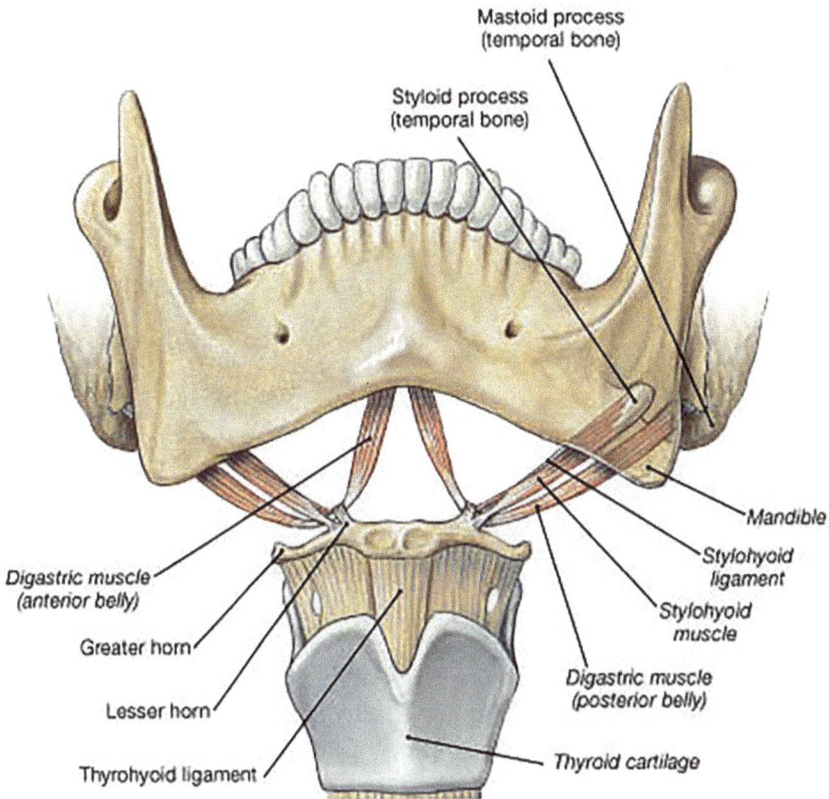

Mastoid process
(temporal bone)

Styloid process
(temporal bone)

Mandible

Stylohyoid
ligament

Stylohyoid
muscle

Digastric muscle
(posterior belly)

Digastric muscle
(anterior belly)

Greater horn

Lesser horn

Thyrohyoid ligament

Thyroid cartilage

(a) Anterior view

It is one of the great pieces of anatomical engineering. The digastric muscle, originating lateral to the styloid process, passes through a slit in the stylohyoid muscle close to its insertion of the hyoid bone then through a fibrinous loop attached to the hyoid bone and continues medially and superiorly to its attachment on the mandible.

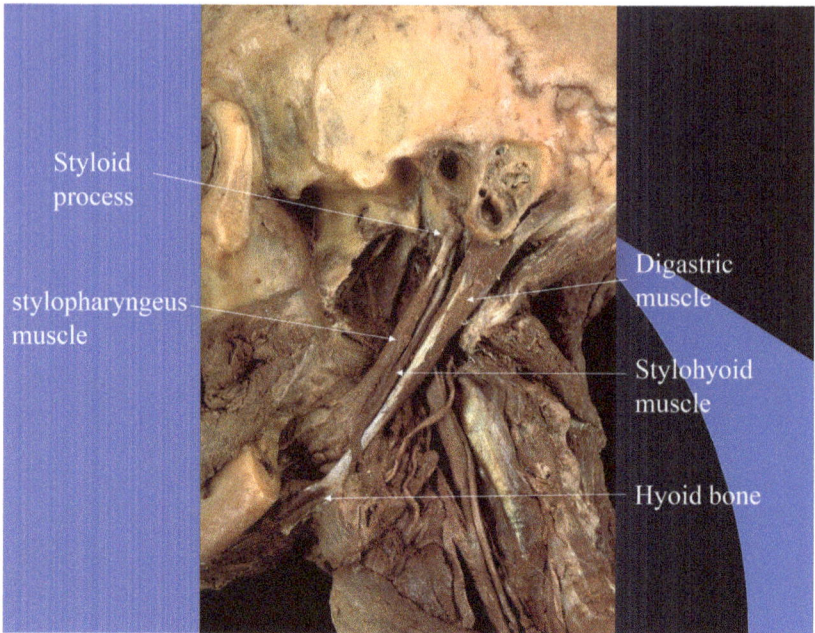

A dissection showing the digastric muscle going through
the stylohyoid muscle and the hyoid bone. Used with permission
of the Willard/Carreiro Collection

The stylohyoid muscles work together like a pair of reins on a horse. As they contract, they pull the hyoid superiorly, thus stabilising it. The infrahyoid muscles, sternohyoid, thyrohyoid and omohyoid stabilise the hyoid inferiorly when they contract.

This stabilisation allows the muscles to the tongue and the mandible to work to their best advantage.

Middle constrictor muscle ⎤
Hyoglossus muscle   ⎥—— Attached to the
Genioglossus muscle   ⎦   greater horn

Chondroglossus muscle ⎤
Stylohyoid muscle   ⎥
Thyrohyoid muscle   ⎥
Geniohyoid muscle   ⎥—— Attached to the body
Omohyoid muscle   ⎥   of the hyoid bone
Mylohyoid muscle   ⎥
Sternohyoid muscle   ⎦

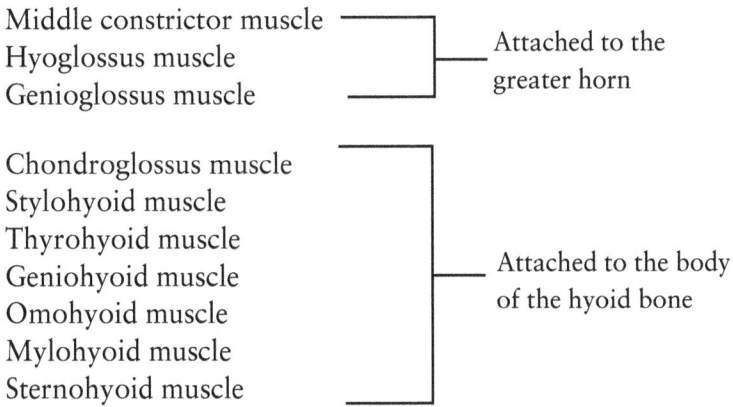

The omohyoid muscle arises from the upper border of the scapula and inserts into the body of the hyoid bone inferiorly, it depresses and stabilises the hyoid bone in the lateral plane. Therefore, when treating the hyoid bone, you have to think laterally, out of the box, and examine the scapula, which in turn is attached to the pelvis via the latissimus dorsi muscle. So, you have to think globally because you will probably have to work on the sacrum to gain an effective result.

It is essential to understand how the hyoid works. It is a little bone and its attachments allow the oropharynx to change pressure and act as a pump.

When treating the auditory tube, you can use all the techniques at your disposal where you think appropriate.

Earlier, when discussing the speed reducers, I described how to release the palatine bone and realign it in the grooves of the pterygoid plate. This allows the palatine aponeurosis more flexibility and therefore better pressure change.

Also, you will have to release the zygoma and the vomer pump using the vomer pump technique.

Finally, I would always look at the cranial vertebral junction and pay attention to the drainage through the mediastinum.

No treatment of the auditory tube is complete without releasing and balancing the hyoid bone.

But before you can attend to this little bone it is important that you make sure that the temporal bones are balanced, as is the mandible on the temporal bones, thus you know that the infratemporal muscles are working as efficiently as they can.

I will describe this technique for releasing the hyoid bone for a right-handed person.

Have the patient lying supine and stand on the right side of the patient and with your left hand, palpate the hyoid bone.

Find the angle of the mandible and with your thumb and first finger move your hand inferiorly and medially to palpate the hyoid bone. If you cannot find it get the patient to poke their tongue out and you will feel the hyoid bone move.

Gently hold the hyoid with your finger and thumb.

With your right hand place your middle finger in the sternal notch.

You can then engage the facia of sternohyiod and sternothyroid muscles. Once you have engaged the facia you follow the involuntary mechanism into flexion and extension. In the flexion phase the facia will relax slightly as everything externally rotates and we become shorter and fatter.

As you feel the facia relax, engage it fully and override the mechanism by taking the facia cranially, thus allowing more flexibility within it which allows the hyoid to become free. You will feel it begin to swing around an axis through the body of the hyoid. I personally get the patient to take a few deep breaths and as they do so you will feel the hyoid begin to balance in the midline.

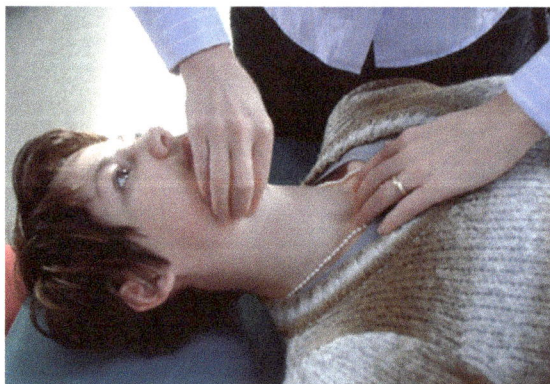

Note the fingers of the left hand with the middle finger in the sternal notch and the right hand palpating the hyoid bone.

However, there is another method of assisting the evacuation of the auditory tube.

This method was shown to me by an ENT surgeon in Russia. Although I know that some of the older American-trained osteopaths used it, over time it seemed to go out of fashion, probably because it is quite invasive. Having said all this, I know it works extremely well, firstly from personal reasons and secondly, from one of my colleagues who had to use it on his son.

The boy, then aged about two years, awoke in the night in acute pain in his ear. My colleague performed the technique on him, which immediately released the pressure. A large amount of detritus effused and the child went back to sleep.

For this technique I have the patient sitting and, if I am working on the right auditory tube, I cradle the head with my left arm and insert a gloved first finger into the mouth as far as the last molar tooth. Anatomically it is impossible to reach the end of the tube, however you can engage the soft palate and push it cranially and laterally towards the opening and in most cases, you will feel through the soft palate a firm cartilaginous ring which is the end of the tube. Push your finger up firmly to the ring and then release quickly, like using a sink plunger to clear a blocked sink, the immediate change in pressure should release the pressure within the tube allowing better evacuation.

In some circles chronic otitis media does not exist over six years of age. However, I have seen children up to the age of twelve showing symptoms of chronic otitis media.

One child was brought to the practice by her mother and for subsequent appointments by her grandmother and accompanied by her younger sister. She was aggressive and very ill mannered, rude to her grandmother and awful to her sister. I treated her for four or five weeks and when I questioned her as to any changes there was only a negative grunt. However, I felt there were changes going on. Finally, one day she came in and again I asked her how she was. A tear developed, and she said "I was frightened to say anything, I began to hear and this week I heard the noise of the gravel as I was walking." She turned to her grandmother and continued "I am so sorry, I know I have been very rude to you all. But I could not hear you."

Summary

Treating the auditory tube and its related problems is one of the finest examples of interrelated osteopathy and the interrelationship of structures.

It is the understanding of the dynamic interface between the body structures, tissue and the physiologic and homeostatic processes necessary for health that makes osteopathy unique.

CHAPTER 6

The Tempo Mandibular and the anterior triangle

The temporo mandibular joint (TMJ) is an uncomplicated structure that can cause considerable pain and discomfort.

The TMJ is a very simple joint. The mandible hangs from a sulcus in the temporal bone and is held in place by a strong capsule.

Within the joint is an articular disc which fits into the sulcus on the temporal bone, this sulcus accommodates the articular surface of the mandible. The disc helps stabilise the condyle within the articular fossa during movement of the mandible.

The mandible is held in place by some powerful ligaments including the stylomandibular ligament and the sphenomandibular ligament and a number of powerful muscles.

Firstly, we have the two pterygoid muscles.

The lateral pterygoid muscle has two heads, the first from the infratemporal surface of the greater wing of the sphenoid and inserts into the fibrous capsule and the articular disc, with the second from the lateral surface of the lateral pterygoid plate and inserts into the neck of the mandible.

The muscle's main role is to pull the capsule clear to stop it impinging on the sternocleidomastoid muscle and the parotid gland as the mandible is depressed.

Depression of the mandible occurs when the digastric muscles, geniohyoid muscles and mylohyoid muscles contract.

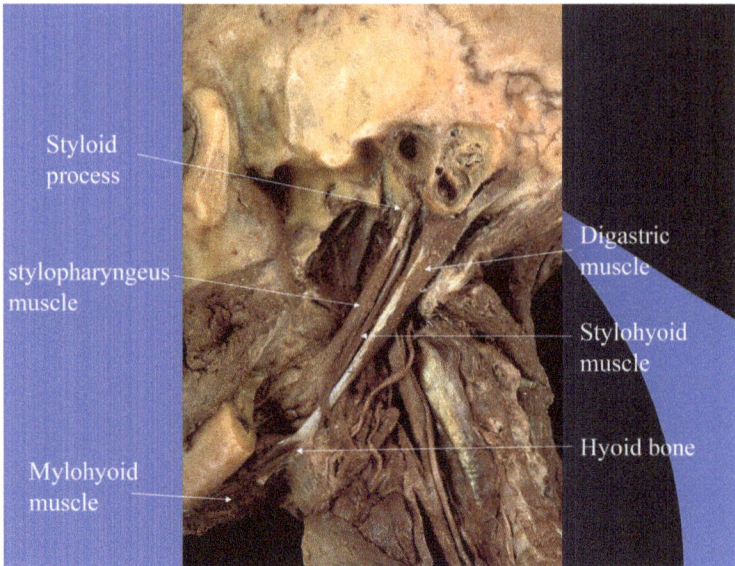

Showing both bellies of digastric muscle,
the hyoid and mylohyoid muscle.
Used with permission of the Willard/Carreiro collection

Elevation or closure is activated by the temporalis muscle, medial pterygoid muscle and the masseter muscle.

The posterior fibres of the temporalis muscle will pull the head of the mandible backwards and the disc is pulled back by the elastic fibres tethering the disc to the temporal bone.

The medial pterygoid muscle arises from the medial aspect of the pterygoid plate of the sphenoid and inserts into the medial aspect of the angle of the mandible. The prime role of this muscle is to elevate the mandible. I always find it fascinating that in anatomy you often get two muscles working together and this is the case with the medial pterygoid and the masseter muscle. The masseter muscle arises from a thick tendinous aponeurosis from the zygomatic arch and inserts into the ramus of the mandible.

These two muscles elevate the mandible with some considerable force.

As osteopaths, we are often called upon to treat this joint for disfunction or pain, and it always amazes me how successful osteopathic treatment can be in alleviating the symptoms and restoring function.

Many times, patients have asked, "can you do something about my bite as I keep catching my tongue?" By working on the associated musculature, balancing the temporal bones, the mandible, hyoid and beyond, one can have a profound effect and restore function.

There are many reasons that the TMJ malfunctions.

It can be due to orthodontic, orthopaedic or occlusive factors. There can be changes in neuromuscular control or psycho-emotional factors. Patients undergoing a great deal of stress for whatever reason often clench or grind their teeth. This causes tension in the surrounding musculature and beyond which can result in pain around the joint and the intimate muscles such as temporalis, masseter and the pterygoid muscles. Other symptoms can include discomfort and headaches often arising from the cervical muscles and their attachments.

Changes in the cranium through basic patterns and strains affecting the membrane can cause changes in movement of the temporal bones and the mandible.

Pain in the TMJ can also be due to bruxism, malocclusion and persistent gum chewing.

One of the common symptoms of TMJ disfunction is a headache. 80 per cent of those presenting have headaches and 40 per cent have facial pain, sometimes confused in differential diagnosis with trigeminal neuralgia. Ear pain, dizziness plus a fullness or ringing in the ears are also quite common symptoms.

The other problem that we as osteopaths are regularly called on to treat are patients who have had braces fitted to correct malalignment of the teeth that have become crowded, crooked or are protruding. Thus, correcting the bite and allowing the top and bottom teeth to meet perfectly.

As a result of these braces to either the upper or lower teeth, the patients often suffer from discomfort and pain.

Osteopathic treatment of patients having braces allows a faster resolution to what the braces are trying to achieve.

All my granddaughters have had braces fitted and one orthodontist commented that he had never seen treatment resolve so quickly and that osteopathic treatment sped up the resolution by up to fifty per cent.

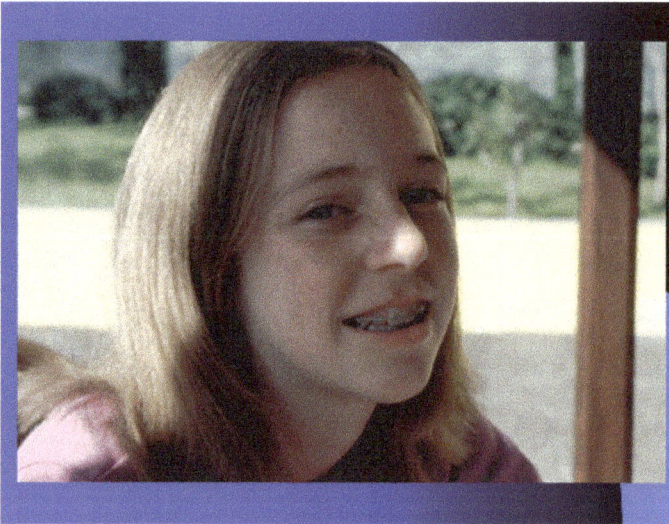

Let us, for a moment, consider the effect on the involuntary mechanism of putting wire around the upper teeth, thus preventing the involuntary movement of internal and external rotation of the maxillae to take place.

As we have seen earlier, the maxillae have no direct contact with the sphenoid which is driving the movement. Movement is conveyed via the speed reducers, the zygoma, the palatine and the vomer.

The sphenoid and the speed reducers will struggle to move the maxillae in the flexion and extension phases and this will cause tension within the mechanism and the membrane. Some of people with braces have no symptoms at all but those that do have side effects which can include headaches, facial pain and feelings of discomfort within the mouth. However, I have also seen patients showing symptoms of stomach pains, nausea and other varied somatic visceral symptoms associated with the vagus nerve (cranial nerve X) that were not apparent pre-braces and have only developed since the braces have been in place.

I was asked to treat a young girl of twelve years of age. Prior to having braces fitted on both her upper and lower teeth she was a fit happy young girl with very few cares in the world. However, following the fitting of the braces she began to get pains in her head and a few weeks later she developed pains in her stomach associated with nausea. Her parents had taken her to her doctor who examined her fully and, finding no apparent reason for the symptoms, put them down to growing pains and her beginning menstruation.

I examined her and found that the mechanism was compromised in such a way that the movement of flexion and extension was minimal. The membrane felt very tight and movement of the temporal bones, the zygoma and the maxillae was negligible.

My treatment consisted in improving and balancing the facial bones and balancing the membrane. I also paid attention to the basiocciput, releasing the occipito-atlantal joint working all the way down to the sacrum. I saw her three times and on the third occasion she reported that all the abdominal symptoms and head pains had eased.

I have always found in cases of symptoms caused by having braces fitted that the key component is the lack of movement of the zygoma. Once this has been freed, by lifting it out of its articulation with the temporal bone at the zygomatic arch, the mechanism begins to resolve. Then by applying treatment to the palatines and the vomer, some form of mobility is restored.

By treating patients with these symptoms using osteopathic techniques to take the stress away from the mechanism and especially the speed reducers, symptoms are often alleviated, improving the patient's well-being.

When treating the TMJ I will use any of the techniques previously described to free the speed reducers, especially the zygoma, in combination with applying my treatment elsewhere in the body.

You will have to balance the temporal bones and then once this is complete you can balance and adjust the mandible.

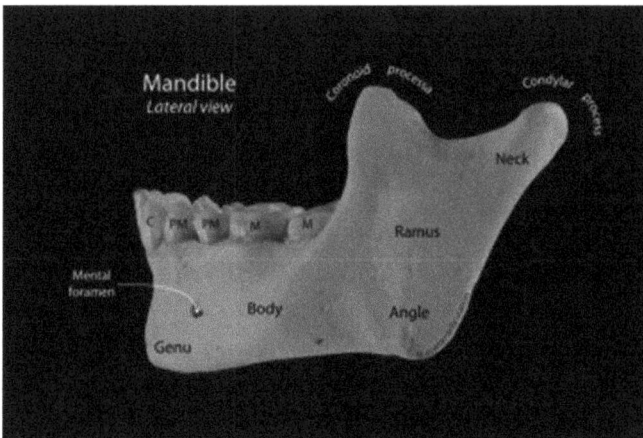

Remember that the mandible is shaped like an angle bracket hanging from the sulcus of the temporal bone.

There are a lot of muscles attached to it as well as the pterygoid muscles. There are the masseter muscles, the buccinator, temporalis, orbicularis oris muscle around the mouth as well as depressor anguli oris and zygomaticus major which blends in with it at the corner of the mouth. All these muscles, at the front of the face, below the eye and to the mouth tend to blend in with each other.

Inferiorly you have the hyiodeus muscles, mylohyoid and geniohyoid plus the anterior belly of the digastric as well as genioglossus from the tongue. The platysma is attached to the inferior border of the mandible.

When you are balancing the mandible, you have to take these muscles into account as well as the fact that we consider it to be two bones, as is the frontal bone, joined at the symphysis menti.

The mandible is very mobile. It can close against the upper teeth in the maxilla or open wide to eat or yawn. It can also move laterally within the bounds of its articulation with the temporal bone and this is where the problems often arise, which are due to this sideways movement.

Having balanced the temporal bones, we can now balance the mandible.

Take a comfortable position at the head of the patient and relax. Have good listening posts with your forearms supported on the table then allow your fingers to alight onto the mandible with the little finger, digit five, on the angle of the mandible. Rest the other fingers along the body of the mandible ensuring that you are not underneath it as you could get drawn inferiorly by the fascia of the platysma.

You can now engage the mechanism. Feel the mandible externally rotate as the angle of the mandible widens and moves inferiorly pivoting around the symphysis menti. You can now begin to balance the mandible in the midline. Like all balancing techniques you will feel everything relax and become very calm before entering another phase of movement.

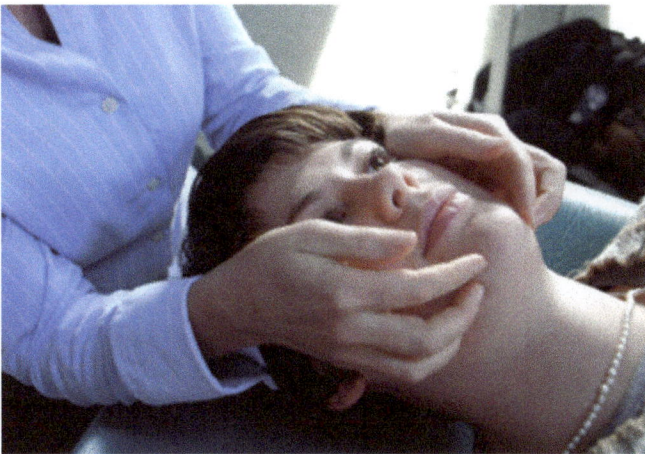

Note how the fingers are spread along the mandible.

To successfully treat problems with the TMJ you have to look at the complete structure. Not only can the muscles activating movement of the TMJ be part of the problem but you have to consider looking further afield. The cervical and thoracic paravertebral muscles can have an adverse effect by causing stress and strains through the occiput therefore affecting the temporal bone and the parietals. Conversely the anterior triangle, the hyoid bone, the clavicle and the platysma can also have an adverse effect on the movement of the TMJ.

However, many structures below the TMJ can cause changes of movement.

Reflect on how changes at sacral/pelvic level can affect the TMJ via the facial links from the psoas muscle inserted into the medial aspect of the superior part of the femur and arising from the transverse processes of the lumbar vertebrae, through the respiratory diaphragm where the facia invaginates with that of the superior aspect of the diaphragm the superiorly on the pericardial fascia, the pretrachael fascia to the cranial base where it can affect movement.

This is what I term global osteopathy. A.T. Still often treated areas far removed from the site of the pain to obtain relief and I find it sad that some osteopaths are very narrow in their approach and if they had better peripheral vision, I am sure they would be surprised at the results they could achieve.

When in practice with colleagues who were finding a problem difficult or when students find themselves unable to find a way forward, I always get them look elsewhere and often by applying your skill to other areas you get the result you require.

CHAPTER 7

Trigeminal Neuralgia

Before the advent of aspirin, trigeminal neuralgia was acknowledged to be the biggest cause of suicide in northern Europe.

It is a compression neuropathy giving prolonged severe pain for considerable periods.

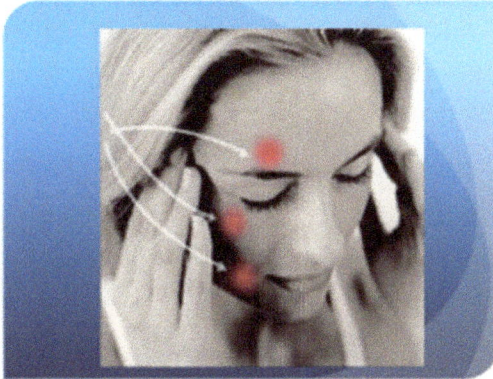

It can also be less intense giving a pricking feeling which can be constant.

As the trigeminal nerve supplies is sensory to the dura mater, it can also present as deep head pain and is something that should be taken into account in the differential diagnosis of headaches and head pain.

The pathogenesis is such that there is nerve root compression usually of vascular origin, and there is inflammatory demyelination of the nerve root which is often associated with ephaptic conduction of surrounding fibres and spinal trigeminal nucleus facilitation.

The possible causes are compression of the rostral and anterior portion of the superior cerebellar artery, which will give second and third division pain, and compression of the caudal and posterior portion of the anterior inferior cerebellar artery.

The other causes can be from aneurysm, meningioma in the cerebellopontine angle, from trauma following a road traffic accident or serious blow to the cranium.

The persistent compression will cause local demyelination and this can lead to axonal degeneration.

The trigeminal nerve is the largest of the cranial nerves and even in the developing foetus you can see it standing out as early as 36 days.

It is the longest cranial nerve and is two thirds sensory and one third motor.

It is sensory to the skin of the scalp/face/mouth/teeth nasal cavity and the paranasal sinuses.

The motor component supplies the muscles of mastication, tensor veli palatini, tensor tympani, the anterior body of the digastric muscle and mylohyoid muscle.

The nerve is divided into three divisions.

The first division is the ophthalmic division (Cr N V1) which exits through the superior orbital fissure.

It is sensory only via the lacrimal, frontal and nasociliary nerves.

This division also supplies the cornea, the skin of the forehead, the scalp, eyelids and nose plus the mucous membranes of the paranasal sinuses and the nasal cavity.

The second division, the maxillary division (Cr N V2) exits through the foramen rotundum and is sensory to the skin of the face over the maxilla and upper lip. It is also sensory to the upper teeth via the superior alveolar nerve, the mucous membrane of the nose, the maxillary air sinuses and the palate.

The third division is the largest, the mandibular division (Cr N V3). It exits through the foramen ovale and is both sensory and motor.

The sensory division supplies the skin of the cheek and mandible, the side of the head and the teeth of the lower jaw via the inferior alveolar nerve, the temporomandibular joint, the mucous membrane of the mouth and the anterior two thirds of the tongue.

The motor division supplies all the muscles of mastication, mylohyoid muscle, the anterior belly of digastric muscle, tensor veli palatini muscle and tensor tympani.

The pain distribution of trigeminal neuralgia is 44 per cent maxillary division, 36 per cent mandibular division and 20 per cent ophthalmic division.

When confronted with a possible case of trigeminal neuralgia you have to consider your differential diagnosis.

The main ones to take into consideration are neoplasms, vascular malformation of the brain stem, vascular insult and in younger people multiple sclerosis. Finally, postherpetic pain in the first division is possible especially if there is an antecedent rash and possible scarring.

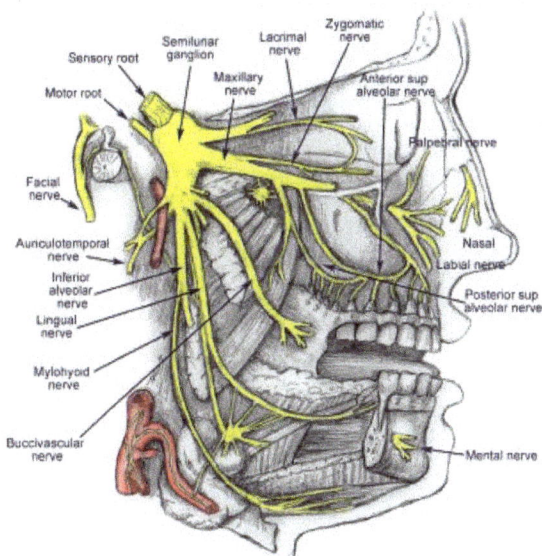

Distribution of the trigeminal nerve.

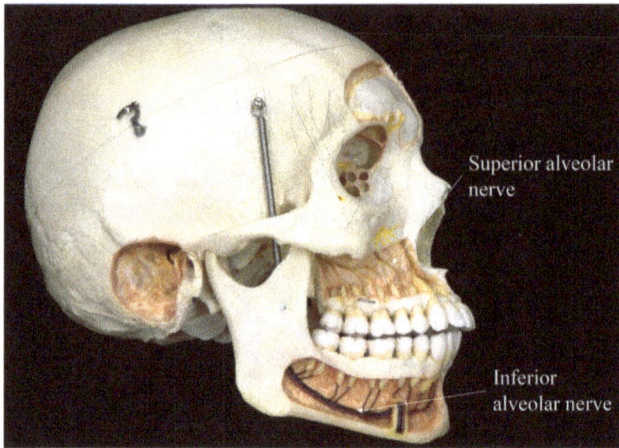

A skull showing the nerves to the teeth.
Used with permission of the Willard/Carreiro Collection

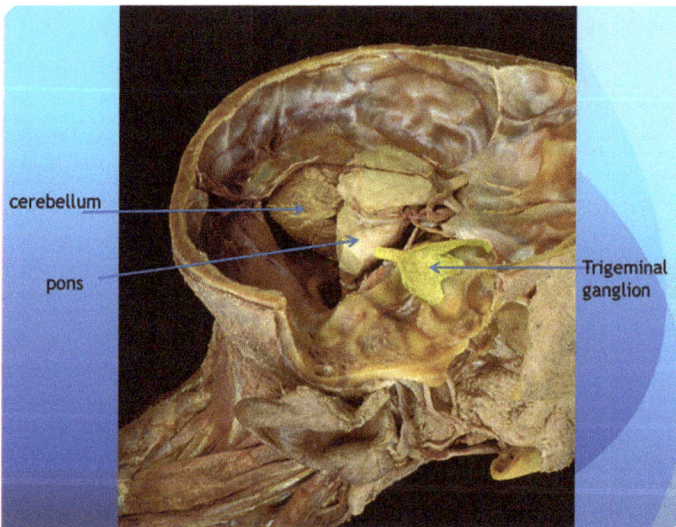

A dissection showing the trigeminal ganglion lying in
Meckel's cave which is formed by two layers of the dura
mater near the petrous portion of the temporal bone.
Used with permission of the Willard/Carreiro Collection

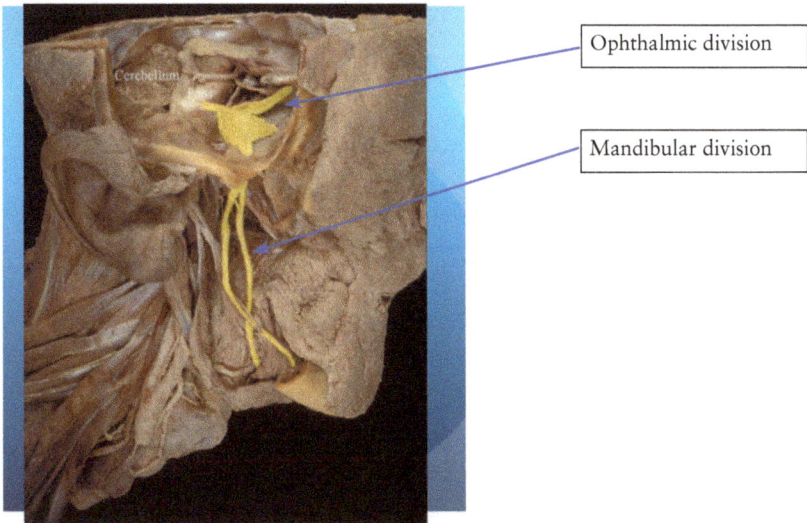

The route of the ophthalmic division and
the mandibular division of the trigeminal nerve.
Used with permission of the Willard/Carreiro Collection

Over the years I have treated many cases of trigeminal neuralgia and have found that you have to apply yourself to evaluating and treating areas of the face that are not functioning properly.

This is especially true of the zygoma where its altered and compromised movement is often the key to why the temporal bone is not moving as it should. You should also look more further afield. Changes in altered mobility and compromised movement are often caused by changes in the pelvis and sacrum and the lower extremities.

You can use any of the techniques described in this book. However, I do find myself invariably lifting the frontal bone and the parietal bones at the beginning of treatment to give more space.

As well as working on the face I also apply myself to looking at the membrane, especially the infratentorial part towards the foramen magnum.

This area around the pons and the foramen magnum is very congested; there are a number of nerves and blood vessels and a lot of fluid all crammed into a small space.

Ann Wales, that great American osteopath who had worked with Sutherland, always maintained that after a general anaesthetic the brain stem seems to be pulled down further into the foramen magnum, giving headaches and other symptoms and I feel the same happens in cases of trigeminal neuralgia.

To attempt to relieve these symptoms I lift the membrane, especially around the foramen, to give more space.

To do this I take a hold under the occiput, engage the membrane and follow the falx cerebelli inferiorly to the foramen magnum. Once there I observe with my hands and then proceed to lift or suck the brain stem cranially.

This, in conjunction with working on the facial bones, seems to have a relieving effect.

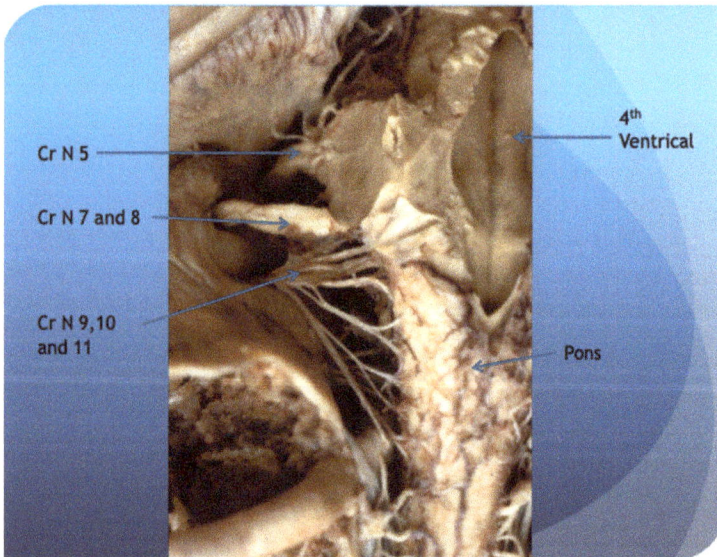

Used with permission of the Willard/Carreiro Collection

CHAPTER 8

The Sinuses

How many times do we see patients complaining of pain over the sinuses, especially the maxillary sinus? I often used to get patients referred to me by a dentist where the patient had presented with pain in the upper molars and on examination the teeth were found to be fine, but the pain persisted and the problem was found to be in the maxillary sinus. Anatomically the root of the tooth can penetrate through the floor of the sinus. This phenomenon is often asymptomatic but other times can cause intense pain.

The paranasal sinuses are rudimentary at birth and grow steadily until early adult life, although the maxillary sinus continues to grow very slowly into old age; this is why the face elongates in the older person.

There are many interesting things written about the function of the paranasal sinuses. They add resonance to the voice and give lightness to the cranium, some feel that they give strength to certain areas within the skull.

There are six paranasal sinuses. We have already discussed one of them, the auditory tube and the others are the maxillary, the frontal, the sphenoidal, the ethmoidal and the mastoid, which drains into the middle ear and is eventually vacated via the auditory tube.

The sinus cavities are lined with a mucosal blanket of pseudostratified columnar epithelium that is ciliated. It contains muco glycoproteins, immunoglobulins and inflammatory cells.

There are two layers, the first the serous or sol layer contains cilia and an outer viscous layer, a gel layer, that is exposed to the environment and which traps particulate matter.

This matter or detritus is moved by a low energy movement where the cilia beat in random motion but in the same direction. It is in this way that the sinuses drain into the nasal cavity.

There are a number of factors that affect the viscosity within the sinus.

Inflammation, cystic fibrosis, viruses, bacterial infections and anticholinergic medication can cause viscosity changes. Also, some foods containing histamine, for instance alcohol, some dairy foods, wheat, eggs and fish, can all affect the viscosity and therefore the movement of fluid within the sinus.

Acute sinusitis is mainly caused by viruses, bacteria or fungal pathogens.

The most common site of acute sinusitis is the maxillary sinus often as a complication of a rhinovirus infection.

The main defining symptom is that the pain is affected by gravity, thus it is worse by day and better by night. The pain is caused by pressure over the thinnest part of the bone.

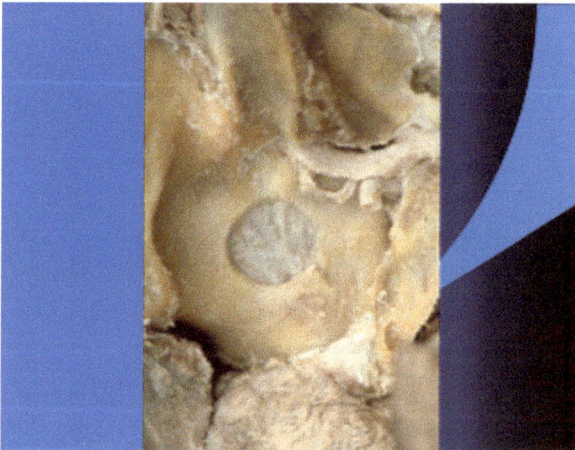

Dissection showing the thin bone of the maxillary sinus.
Used with permission of the Willard/Carreiro collection

Chronic sinusitis is also mostly common in the maxillary antrum. It is a dull, aching, gnawing pain often associated with a tired ipsilateral eye pain, there can also be persistent headaches and ocular changes.

When presented with a patient with chronic sinusitis, you have to consider in your differential diagnosis the possibility of a mucocele or even osteomyelitis (Pott's disease) in the frontal/occipital component, with localised pain, swelling and erythematous forehead peau d'orange skin changes.

The Maxillary Sinus

This sinus is one large cavity anatomically. It is present at birth and grows rapidly for the first three years of life and then slows down until the eruption of the teeth.

Clinically it can present in the first year of life, however the maxilla in the infant is almost square in shape and as the child grows the maxilla becomes higher and longer and although it seems to stop growing in middle life it actually continues to elongate as we get older.

The nerve supply is from the anterior and posterior alveolar nerves, which are branches of the trigeminal nerve.

The blood supply is from the facial, infraorbital and palatine arteries and it is drained through the maxillary cistern via the ethmoidal infundibulum.

The Frontal Sinus

This sinus is normally one cavity over each orbit.

At birth this sinus is a very small slit-like area above the nasal bones. The sinus actually arises out of the anterior ethmoid group of sinuses.

At the end of the second year of life it invades the vertical portion of the frontal bone and until the age of four the antrum is very thin, spreading laterally towards the orbital rim by the age of ten.

The symptoms from this sinus are clinically reported from seven to eight years of age.

Again, the nerve supply is via a branch of the trigeminal nerve, via the supraorbital branches of the ophthalmic nerve, and its blood supply is from the supraorbital and anterior ethmoidal arteries.

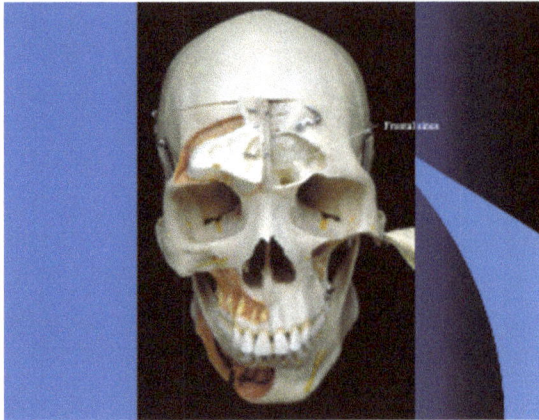

Slide showing the large frontal sinus which drains inferiorly
through the frontonasal duct.
With permission of the Willard/Carreiro collection

The Ethmoidal Sinus

As we have seen previously the ethmoid is a very delicate light bone that can cause quite severe symptoms. Remember that is attached to the falx cerebri thus it can affect the way the membrane is working.

This sinus is made up of four to seventeen small cavities each side of the midline.

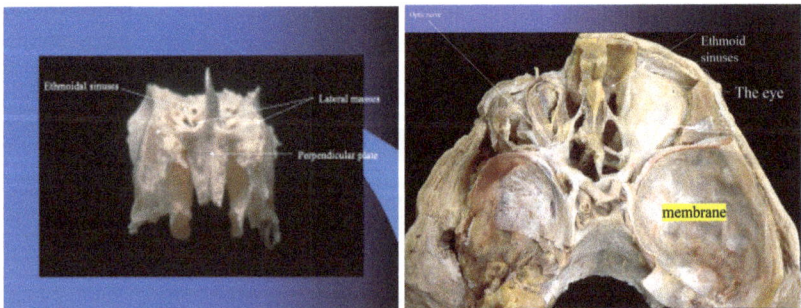

The ethmoid sinuses.
Used with permission of the Willard/Carreiro Collection

The ethmoid sinus is almost fully developed at birth and reaches adult size by twelve years of age, it also can present clinically within the first year of life. There is sometimes inflammation of the sinus via an orbital cellulitis which transfers through the very thin, fine bony tissue of the lateral masses.

The nerve supply is via the sphenopalatine ganglion with the anterior and posterior ethmoidal nerve and the orbital branch of the ganglion.

The blood supply is from the sphenopalatine and ethmoidal arteries.

These three sinuses all present with pain over the sinus but however, our next sinus the sphenoidal sinus presents with vertex pain due to its trigeminal nerve supply. There can also be throbbing pain behind the eyes and some ocular pressure.

The sphenoidal sinus is usually one large sinus divided asymmetrically by a midline partition.

It is supplied by the maxillary and ethmoidal nerves and the blood supply is from the posterior ethmoidal artery.

During the first year of life it begins to develop and it presents clinically from age of three years.

When you are presented with a case where you think it might be a sphenoidal sinus problem consider also a possible complication from a cavernous sinus thrombosis or a tumour within the sinus.

Over the years I have pondered on the best way of treating sinus problems especially chronic sinusitis.

One year I was in Maine in the USA and listened to a lecture by the most amazing osteopath called Anne Wales. As I have said previously, she worked with Sutherland and all those great pioneering osteopaths. She had the most wonderful hands and her skill and application of applied anatomy were the best I have ever come across.

She said that to treat the sinuses she followed a routine.

Now, most osteopaths follow what the body tells them and they do not have a definitive routine, but Anne did. So here it is.

1   Observe the coronal suture and if caught lift the frontals off.
2   Widen and narrow the ethmoidal notch.
3   Release the frontosphenoid articulation.
4   Balance and adjust the zygomatic bones.
5   Release the perpendicular plate of the vomer and ethmoid (vomer pump.)
6   Adjust the palatine bones in relation to the pterygoid process.
7   Adjust the spheno-squamous and petro-sphenous articulations.
8   Release the cranio-vertebral junction.
9   Stimulate the spheno-palatine ganglion.

CHAPTER 9

The Sacrum

When I was a student and we came to discuss the sacrum, it was in the context of the lumbo-sacral joint, the sacroiliac joint and that it formed one of the primary skeletal curves.

There was no mention of the dural membrane being attached to the second sacral segment and there was a brief reference to the coccyx which we were told hangs off the most caudal segment.

We were taught how to spring the sacroiliac joint, how to mobilise the joint in different directions and how to gap the lumbo-sacral joint and how to spring the joint to increase flexion. All very important for a budding osteopath to treat the plethora of musculoskeletal problems which would come his way.

Then one weekend, whilst in my final year, I was invited to a seminar by a lady osteopath who trained in the United States of America.

The topic of the seminar was the sacrum and I went because I was expecting to find other ways of attending to these musculoskeletal problems, what I did not expect was to be told how important the sacrum was in maintaining homeostasis within the human body.

That the sacrum was a springboard, the centre of a spider's web that linked the lower extremities and the pelvis to the upper body. I learned how the sacrum helped maintain the integrity of the pelvic bowl and all that was contained within that basket. It was a revelation to me, but I felt very limited in how to work and treat this triangular bone and all its applied anatomy.

The sacrum really is a quite amazing structure.

When I was teaching at what was then the British School of Osteopathy, I found a box containing about forty or fifty sacra. The fascinating thing was they were all different. While some were very light to hold, others felt like a brick, and where some were flat, some were concave and some convex. Some were quite thin, others very thick and had an immense density to them. Obviously, some were male and some female, there were no children's sacra but the interesting thing is that they all performed the same anatomical job for that human being. They were all perfect and there were no malformations. So, when you put your hand under a sacrum, feel what it is like; it is living, breathing human tissue.

It took me until I began my quest for the involuntary mechanism to fully realise what my American lady was saying and how important the sacrum is and what an enigmatic structure it is.

So, when you palpate the sacrum, what does it feel like? Is it hard, is it moving, does it float, is it breathing?

Palpation is your life tool, refine it. Sutherland said you have ten all-seeing thinking eyes and as well as using your fingers, use the whole hand. When palpating a sacrum have one hand under the sacrum and the other on the abdomen or the thoraco-lumbar junction so that you feel between your hands, in three dimensions?

If you have small hands or the patient is heavy, you do not have to have them supine because the weight may stop you feeling, so turn the patient on their side and you can feel just the same. You have to be able to modify techniques to suit you.

Think of the spider's web and the sacrum being in the centre. Piriformis muscle originates from the sacrum, the lower lumbar vertebrae and the capsule of the sacroiliac joint, it then exits the pelvis through the greater sciatic foramen and inserts into the greater trochanter of the femur. So, the sacrum now has a direct relationship with the femur, the facia surrounding it also invaginates with other facias around the hip joint and the muscles from the lower extremity.

High up on the medial aspect of the femur is the insertion of the psoas muscle. This muscle works as a hip flexor in conjunction with the iliacus muscle which is inserted on the femur just above the psoas.

The iliacus arises from the iliac fossa and joins with the psoas major muscle working as major hip flexors. However, they also convey a fascial chain from the lower extremity through the pelvis superiorly along the lumbar vertebrae under the medial arcuate ligament of the diaphragm with also the quadratus lumborum muscle which enters the mediastinum by passing under the lateral arcuate ligament. These two muscles convey a facial chain to the superior aspect of the diaphragm and as the pericardial sac is adhered to the superior aspect this fascial chain proceeds cranially from the precardiac fascia to the pretrachael fascia and thus to the cranial base.

Posteriorly the sacroiliac ligaments coalesce with the Sacro tuberous ligament which then coalesces with the long head of the biceps fermoris muscle, which originates from the ischial tuberosity and is attached to the head of the fibula. Therefore, there is a fascial chain from the lower leg and foot superiorly to the posterior aspect of the pelvis and sacrum which then coalesces with the sacral fascial raphe extending onto the posterior lumber fascia which will then go cranially to the cervical fascia and the base of the occiput.

In the middle of all this is the sacrum, a key part of the chain, the centre of the spider's web.

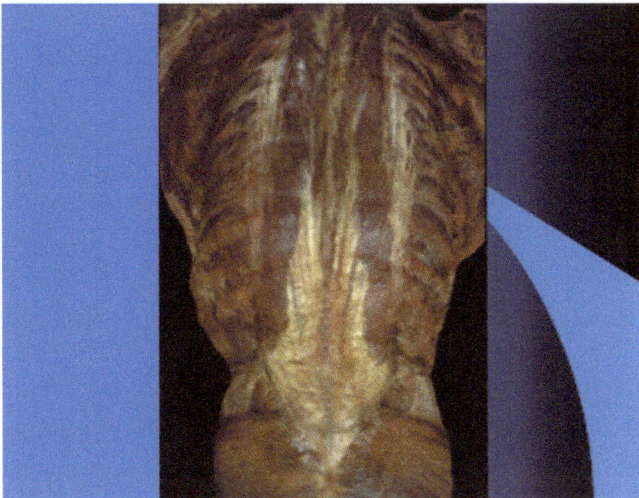

Posterior Sacro-lumbar fascia extending superiorly.
Used with permission of the Willard/Carreiro collection

The sacrum also plays a major part in how the pelvic floor works and its integrity.

The pelvic floor is a basket of muscle which basically holds up the contents of the abdominal cavity. The main muscle is the levator ani which is often divided into various components, Iliococcygeus, pubo-rectalis, and pubococcygeus. The levator ani muscle is attached to the sacrum by the anterior sacral coccygeal ligament.

This strong but thin layer of muscles holds up the contents of the abdominal waste disposal components and the reproductive organs.

There is however a considerable amount of body fluid within the pelvic cavity as well as fatty sinuses and movement helps this fluid to remain healthy. Once movement slows or stops the pelvic cavity becomes unhealthy, stasis occurs and the contents of the floor suffer as a consequence.

I have noticed over the years that people who ride horses have far fewer problems in the pelvic bowl than those who do not and I put this down to the constant movement that takes place when riding straddling a horse this gives rise to pressure changes within the pelvic bowl allowing a good fluid exchange.

It is essential that firstly the pelvic floor muscles are as strong as can be and secondly that there is a good interchange of fluid within the pelvic bowl, and an improved blood supply and drainage. Horse riding allows that change of pressure that results in improved homeostasis.

For those that do not ride, we have to devise exercises and techniques to strengthen the floor and improve fluid exchange, one of these techniques is a pelvic lift, which I think was first devised by Sutherland.

With the patient lying on their side, I stand facing them and with my right hand I palpate the ischial tuberosity. I then move my fingers medially to find a soft area called the ischial-rectal fossa; this is quite medial to the tuberosity, so as you slide your fingers round the tuberosity you can easily find this soft area.

Now having a flat hand and keeping it firm, you push your fingers into the fossa; it will feel squidgy and soft, especially in those whose pelvic floor has lost its tonicity.

I place my other hand on the patient's back and ask them to breathe in and then breathe out. As they breathe out you will feel the pelvic floor relax, so push your fingers in firmly until there is resistance. Complete this exercise three or four times, on the last one, tell the patient to take a deep breath, hold it and push downwards (I tell ladies to bear down.)

Feel what is happening with your fingers; you should feel the facia resolving and slightly soften and when you feel that the tissue is resolving ask the patient to expel the breath forcibly and you will feel your fingers go further into the bowl.

The changes that take place are quite profound, especially with the fluid in the pelvic bowl sinuses and the fascia.

I used this technique on my wife when she was having problems with the pelvic floor and possible prolapse. I discussed it with her gynaecologist and after six weeks of my treating her every other day he said he had never seen such a change in the integrity of the pelvic floor, so no need for surgery!

We cannot leave this area without talking about the coccyx. If we had one, this is where our tail would be. It is formed of three, four or five segments, the upper segments do not tend to unite until about thirty years of age, but the lower segments tend to fuse together earlier.

The coccyx is usually concave, although they can be quite flat and even convex. The later causes problems giving birth because as the coccyx is protruding into the area of the birth canal the face of the baby is pulled along it, dragging it backwards as in a face presentation.

However, most of the problems arise through trauma and some through child birth.

Older patients have coccygeal problems because they often lose weight and sit for long periods which can give rise to coccygeal pain.

Over the years I have treated many patients with coccygeal pain and over the last twenty-five years I have only had to recourse to treating per rectum once as there is a much better way.

The coccyx is held by the muscle pubococcygeus. It is the medial fibres of the levator ani muscle but distinct in its own right. Pubococcygeus originates from the pubic bone, just under the rim. It runs posteriorly across the pelvic floor to fold round the coccyx like praying hands. It is the muscle that would wag your tail.

This very gentle technique is extremely effective.

If you are right-handed, with the patient lying supine, sit on the left of the patient facing the head. Place your left hand on the pelvic rim with your first finger and thumb either side of the symphysis pubis. Now, take your fingers over the rim, superiorly pushing through the rectus abdominus and engage the pubococcygeus muscle. Your right hand will be under the buttocks and with your middle finger find the tip of the coccyx. Engage the coccyx and the fascia of the pubococcygeus muscle, which often feels like a pair of reins surrounding the coccyx. If you find difficulty in engaging the fascia either gently compress or distract the coccyx and you will feel the mechanism come into play. Find a fulcrum; it will be along the coccyx, usually in the lower third. You can now balance the coccyx with pubococcygeus and wait for the release.

Before I leave this chapter on the sacrum and the pelvis there is however one topic that needs to be covered and that is what you sometimes feel.

Occasionally when you are palpating the sacrum and the membrane the whole of the pelvis feels very tight, almost solid like a very stretched, taut piece of elastic.

To me it feels like it is in shock. If you have ever seen the painting by Edvard Munch called "The Scream" look at it, because this to me this is what the pelvic bowl and membrane feel like.

Having spoken to patients who have exhibited this phenomenon, they often give a story of some form of abuse in both males and females.

About twenty years ago, a lady who worked for me was also a foster mother and she asked me to look at this little girl because she had what she described as a funny-shaped head.

The little girl was six years old. When I put my hand on her head I was forcibly drawn down to the sacrum and pelvis, it was as though I was being pulled down by the fascia.

The lady and I stepped out of the room and I asked her what had happened to this child.

The reply, "she had been abused by her father, uncle and brother since the age of three and that is why she was in foster care."

These cases are all very difficult and have to be handled with great care.

In older patients you can ask some very gentle questions and if they talk to you can advise them re counselling. If it is a child, then if you know the child's doctor you can talk to them and explain that you feel the child is at risk.

Unless you have very firm evidence there is not a lot you can do. What we feel is unique and there are people who will not believe that we can feel these things.

CHAPTER 10

The Eye

The eye is an amazing structure. The eye itself is housed in a very solid bony cave, the orbit, and is extremely fluid both within the eyeball itself and the surrounding housing as well as the vast arterial blood supply and venous drainage. This basically small structure is about one inch in diameter and it is the most used of all our senses. The rod and cone cells of the retina convey information to the brain. The retina has a very substantial blood supply that enters the eye along with the optic nerve in the posterior aspect of the eye in the area known as the optic disc.

This is where, when we are diagnosing and using an ophthalmoscope, we can judge if there is any intercranial pressure as we will see a bulging of the disc.

The bony orbit is made up of seven facial bones. The roof of the orbit is formed by the frontal bone, the posterior part by the greater wing of the sphenoid and a small part of the lesser wing, laterally by the zygoma, which also forms part of the floor of the orbit. The rest of the floor is formed by the maxilla. The medial border is comprised of, anteromedially, the lacrimal bone and posterior to that the ethmoid. Between the frontal and the ethmoid bones posteriorly there is the small triangle of the perpendicular plate of the palatine bone.

Within this bony orbit the eye is protected and cushioned by fat pads and interstitial fluid. This protein rich fluid is constantly being reabsorbed, but views differ as to it going into the lymphatic system which is posterior and adjacent to the orbit.

This fluidity allows the eye to float in the orbit.

The eye itself is composed of the cornea, the anterior chamber containing aqueous humour, a lens suspended by ligaments and a posterior chamber containing vitreous humour.

To move and to hold the eye in place there is a simplistic arrangement of six muscles.

Four of them arise from the common tendinous ring, the optic nerve and vessels pass through this ring, and the four rectus muscles are medial, lateral, inferior and superior.

The other two muscles are the superior and inferior oblique muscles.

The superior oblique muscle arises from the body of the sphenoid and then via a facial loop is attached to the fibrous sheath of the eyeball on its superior aspect. The inferior oblique muscle arises from the floor of the orbit and is inserted into the sclera just behind the coronal equator.

These six muscles move the eyeball in all directions as it floats in the bony orbit.

They are supplied by three different cranial nerves.

Cranial nerve three, the oculomotor, supplies the medial, superior and inferior rectus muscles, inferior oblique muscle and levator palpebrae superioris muscle.

The superior oblique is supplied by cranial nerve four, the trochlear, which is the only cranial nerve to originate from the posterior aspect of the pons.

Finally, cranial nerve six, the abducens, supplies the lateral rectus muscle. This nerve arises from the lateral aspect of the pons and goes under the petro-sphenoid ligament to exit through the superior orbital fissure.

The eye is elliptical in shape and is angled medially towards the optic chiasma.

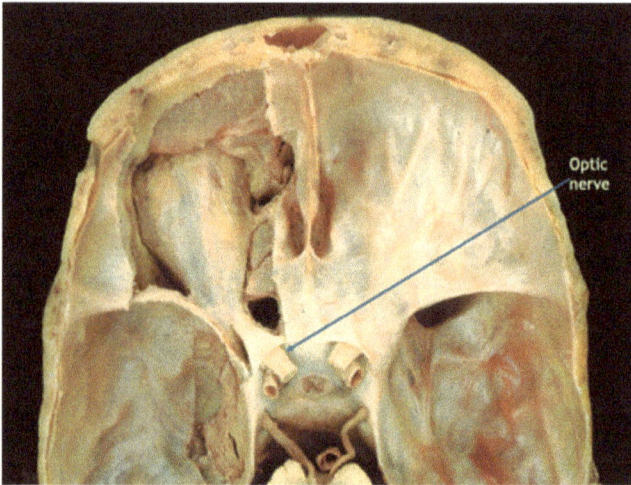

The eye in the bony cranium.
Used with permission of the Willard/Carreiro Collection

Note the angle of the eye; this is very important when you come the examine the eye and treat osteopathically. The eye sits postero-medially in the orbit, so when you put your hands on the eye you will always be taken slightly medially.

The optic nerves cross at the optic chiasma (chiasm from the Greek meaning crossing). The chiasma is situated just above the sella turcica and the diaphragm of sellae. This is clinically significant because when you have visual changes (double vision etc.) in pituitary tumours, as the tumour grows the increase in size causes pressure on the chiasma.

The other interesting fact is that the dural membrane is attached to the ocular ring from where the rectus muscles originate.

This is very easily demonstrated.

Have your colleague or patient sitting comfortably holding a book.

Standing behind them, place your hands on the cranium with a vault hold, your hands will probably cover the parietal bones, the little fingers will be on the squamous temporal.

Make sure your shoulders are relaxed and you are comfortable. Get yourself balanced – find your own Sutherland fulcrum. Then engage the mechanism, palpating the flexion and extension phases. When you are comfortable with this, ask the model to pick up the book and start to read relatively close to the face.

Palpate the movement and when happy with what you feel, ask them to put the book down and look into the distance. Tell them to imagine the mountains and the trees in the far distance, look into infinity, and again just palpate the movement. Feel what it is like, then get them to pick up the book and read again.

What you will notice is a shape change within the membrane. It will tend to go from being wide and fat to being elongated, so why is this?

The rectus muscles of the eye have changed the shape of the eye to accommodate short vision and long vision and infinity. In doing this change in shape has an effect on the common tendinous ring and the dural membrane attached to it.

When you begin to look at the eye osteopathically, you firstly want to observe the movement in the orbital bones.

With your patient lying supine place sit at the head of the table and have your elbows on the table to gain comfortable listening posts.

It is essential when working with the eye that you have soft, gentle hands. You are now in a position to place both hands on the face. Have your thumbs on the frontal bone on glabella. Your hands should comfortably come to rest so that the hypothenar eminence of both hands is just on the spheno-temporal-frontal articulation. Your first finger will come to rest on the nasal bones and from here you can palpate the ethmoid bone. The middle finger should rest on the maxilla and the ring finger on the maxillary-zygomatic articulation.

Finally, the little finger, digit five, will rest on the zygomatic arch.

You now have the bones making up the orbit of the eye under your fingers and hand.

Concentrate on your palpation, feel and examine the movement of each bone in turn. Do the two orbits move in the same way, is there some restriction of some of the bones?

If so, you will have to address this and you may have to disengage some of the sutures, or lift the zygoma and rebalance it with the temporal bone or the maxilla, or you may have to free the palatine bone so that the bony floor of the orbit is moving well in the flexion and extension phases of the movement.

Whatever you find, you must reach a point where the bones of both orbits are moving as well as they can.

Once this is achieved you can now look at the eye itself. Keeping one hand with the fingers around the orbit of the eye put your first, middle and ring fingers together so that the tips of the fingers are together forming a little cave. Ask your patient to close their eyes and gently, as gently as a butterfly landing on a leaf, place these three fingers onto the eyelid.

The little cave formed by the three fingers should just fit over the eyeball.

From here you can palpate in depth, feel what the fluid is like both within and around the eye, remember the socket is lined with fat and interstitial fluid, this allows the eyeball to float within the bony socket. Ask the patient to look up, down and side to side to assess the rectus muscles and the to look at the corners to assess the oblique muscles.

You now have a good idea of how the eye is working in the orbit.

To assist in movement one of the basic techniques you can use is a muscle energy technique on each of the six muscles that work the eye.

It is also quite simple to balance the eye within the bony framework. Once you have attended to the orbit by ensuring all the constituent parts are moving as well as they can, you can then balance the eye itself along a longitudinal axis, anteroposteriorly towards the common tendinous ring.

Another method I use is to slide one hand under the vault so you have the occiput in your hand and then engage the dural membrane. With the other hand take the three finger palpatory hold on the eye. Palpate its movement and then begin to lift the membrane posteriorly and you will feel the orbit move; you can now balance the eye around the tendinous ring using the dural membrane.

All these techniques are of great value when you want to improve the blood supply and the fluidity of the eye. Patients with dry eyes and glaucoma have noticed a benefit when they have been treated osteopathically.

CHAPTER 11

The Shoulder

You may easily ask yourself what has the shoulder go to do with the face?

Well, think about the anatomy of the shoulder, not just the glenohumeral joint but the whole of the shoulder girdle.

In very basic terms the shoulder girdle is slung from the base of the skull by the muscle trapezius and is strapped to the pelvis through the muscle latissimus dorsi and its attachment to the sacrum and the iliac crest through the thoracolumbar fascia.

The latissimus dorsi has fibres attached to the inferior angle of the scapula in over 80 per cent of people.

The only bony configuration the shoulder girdle has is the sternoclavicular joint, otherwise it floats in muscle and fascia.

The glenohumeral joint is by far the most flexible joint in the body, it can elevate 180 degrees, it can rotate 360 degrees and it is supported by some very strong muscles.

The scapula has a shallow sulcus and the joint is really like an angle bracket, i.e. with a back, a top but no sides.

The clavicle is attached to the scapula at the acromioclavicular joint and to the sternum at the sternoclavicular joint and is S-shaped with attachments for the sternocleidomastoid muscle. However, the trapezius muscle is attached to the lateral aspect of the superior surface as is the deltoid muscle. Medially, the pectoralis major is attached to the anterior surface of the clavicle and the subclavius attaches it to the first rib.

So now we have a picture of the trapezius muscle being slung from the occiput and being attached to both the clavicle and the scapula and it is stabilised by being attached to the spinous processes of T4-T12.

The serratus anterior muscle arising from the medial inferior border of the scapula and attaching anteriorly to ribs 1-8 stabilises the scapula in its medial plane.

The rotator cuff muscles, supraspinatus, infraspinatus, teres major, teres minor and subscapularis arise from the scapula and are responsible for rotation and stability within the glenohumeral joint. Other prime movers are the deltoid, triceps (both heads), latissimus dorsi and pectoralis major.

The shoulder girdle fits onto the body of the thorax like a cape. If you release the muscles attaching it to the spine and pelvis and cut the clavicle, the whole of the shoulder girdle will come away.

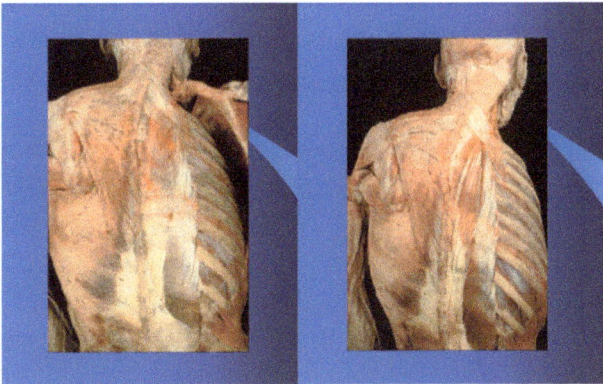

The shoulder girdle removed showing how it is slung from the occiput and attached to the spinous processes. Used with permission of the Willard/Carreiro Collection

Below is a diagram of the structures that form the walls of the axilla. The axilla is basically a triangle with serratus anterior medially, pectoralis major anteriorly and teres major posteriorly, with the head of the humerus being the most lateral part.

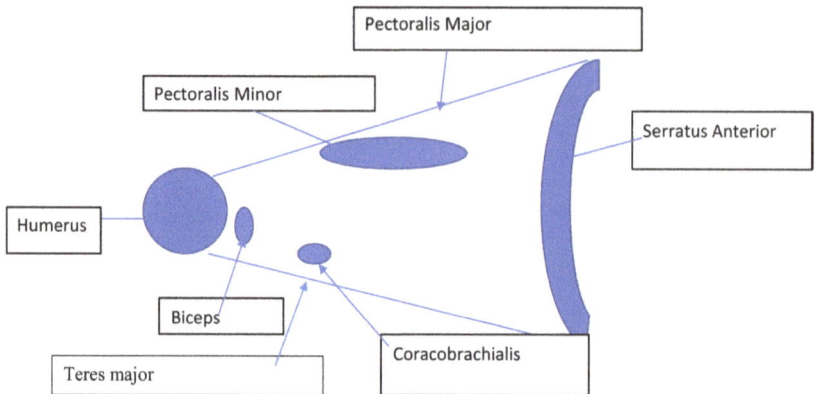

Within this triangle is the joint capsule ligaments
and associated musculature.

Hanging from the inferior border of the clavicle, surrounding subclavius and descending inferiorly is the clavipectoral fascia. It surrounds pectoralis minor and then attaches to the deep fascia of the armpit.

The scapula is also attached to the body of the hyoid bone by the omohyoid muscle which descends inferiorly and laterally to the superior border of the scapula either in or adjacent to the suprascapular notch it is part of the infrahyoid muscle group that depresses the hyoid bone and stabilises it to allow the suprahyoid muscles to work.

This muscle and the sternocleidomastoid muscle will affect the way the anterior triangle of the lower face works.

There are many ways of treating the shoulder, however I will confine myself in just using the involuntary mechanism.

Firstly, balance the scapula. To do this I have the patient supine and sitting at the head I begin with balancing the clavicles. This is not always easy, you should have soft hands and place the fingers along the superior aspect of the clavicle, the digit (little finger) resting on the acromioclavicular joint, the fingers spread along the clavicle with the first finger resting on the sternoclavicular joint. Your thumb will be just under the clavicle.

You now look for a fulcrum, remembering that the clavicle is S-shaped. The fulcrum is normally in the medial half of the bone.

Once the clavicle is balanced you can apply yourself to balancing the scapula.

Slide your hands under the upper body to have the scapula resting in the palms of your hand. Engage the mechanism and you will feel the scapulae float. Find a fulcrum, normally in the upper medial quadrant, and balance around the fulcrum following the movement to a point of ease that refines itself around a single point.

Now you have balanced these two bones, you can begin to think about balancing the glenohumeral joint.

There are three ways that I will balance the glenohumeral joint and the rotator cuff, ligaments, the fluid surrounding the joint and the interstitial fluid.

Let us first consider balancing the humerus with the scapula and clavicle.

With the patient sitting on the treatment table, bring it to the right height so you can place your thumbs over the greater tubercle of the humerus then with one hand spread your fingers along the spine of the scapula and with the other hand your fingers will be along the clavicle.

Now engage the mechanism, feel the scapula and the clavicle externally rotating in the flexion phase and internally rotating in the extension phase. When you are comfortable with this, with your thumbs on the tubercle of the humerus, gently bring your thenar eminences together around the humerus and lift it slightly superiorly further into the joint capsule. As you do so you will feel the humerus, scapula and the clavicle begin to float. You can now balance the humerus with the scapula and clavicle focusing on a midline that is under your thumbs.

The second method I use is, standing to the side of the patient take the same finger holds on the scapula and clavicle then bring your thumbs under the axilla. See the diagram below. Your thumbs should now be under the suspensory ligament which is an inferior extension of the clavipectoral fascia. If you take your thumbs superiorly you will take the tension of the fascia and again feel the whole glenohumeral joint begin to float. As it floats you will be able to balance the ligaments and musculature around a focal point/fulcrum.

Remember there is a lot of fluid within this joint.

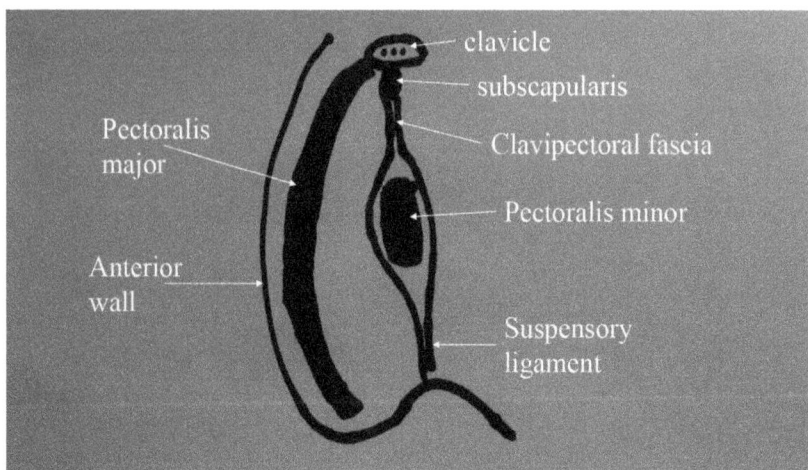

The last method I use is one that patients find very strange. With the patient lying supine place one hand under the glenohumeral joint and the other hand on top. You now have the whole of the joint between your two hands. The patient thinks that you are not doing anything; all they feel is a warmth around the joint.

The object of this technique is to balance and change the fluids within the joint, the intracellular fluid, the extracellular fluid and the interstitial fluid and the synovial fluid. They all feel very different.

Synovial fluid will feel more glutinous, it has a much firmer texture to it.

Interstitial fluid is the fluid that fills the spaces between cells. It is very complex and has neurotransmitters, fatty acids, amino acids, sugars, coenzymes, salts and hormones.

OSTEOPATHY WITHOUT BORDERS

Extracellular fluid has a high concentration of sodium and low potassium, while intracellular fluid is exactly the opposite.

These fluids are very powerful and to increase the potency within them is quite amazing for healing and health in general.

I find that using these techniques, often combining them with some articulatory techniques, is extremely useful. However, I always do the articulation first and then balance the fluids.

CHAPTER 12

The treatment of babies, infants and children

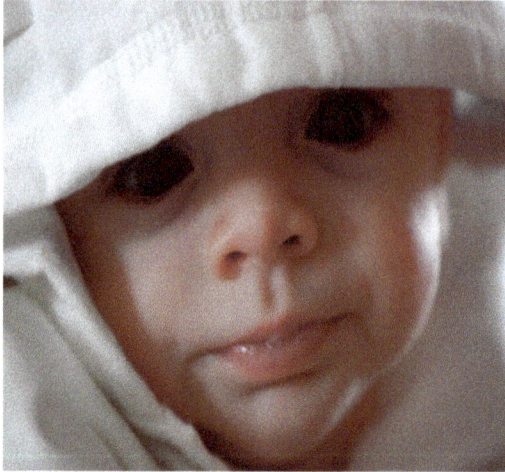

Osteopaths have a long history of treating babies, infants and children and it is extremely rewarding.

William Garner Sutherland stated "Normalizing the structure of the new born head ranks among the most valuable procedures in medicine today. The potential for good in the first few hours of life far exceeds what may be accomplished later."

Andrew Taylor Still wrote about treating children in the 19th century.

Viola Fryman in 1992 wrote about the osteopathic management on neurological development in children, and Beryl Arbuckle wrote a considerable number of texts on the treatment of children especially with cerebral palsy up to her death in 1992.

To treat babies and infants you must have a good knowledge of the physiology and the anatomy, which is very different to that of an adult.

Development of the cranium

The cranium is comprised of two main components, the cranial base and the cranial vault. They are both formed in mesenchyme. If mesenchyme is stretched, membrane is formed, if it is compressed, cartilage is formed.

There are two types of bones within the body: those that develop via endochondral ossification and those that develop via intramembranous ossification.

During endochondral bone development, a cartilaginous template forms preceding ossification. This is used by all the axial bones (vertebral column and ribs) and appendicular bones of the body except part of the clavicle.

The cranial base, sensory capsules and pharyngeal arch cartilages also form via endochondral ossification. (Larsen 4th edition)

Thus, the cranial base formed is formed in cartilage.

The vault is developed as intramembranous ossification from a sheet of membrane that covers the forebrain, which expands as the primitive hemispheres grow and expand below them.

The vault comprises of the parietals, the squama of the occiput (parts between the parietals) the squama of the temporal bone, the edges of the greater wings of the sphenoid and the frontal bone, and it is designed to accommodate growth in the infant and child. The vault adapts to change more than the cranial base.

The cranial base is ossified in cartilage. During the fourth week of intrauterine life the forebrain bends ventrally around the end of the notochord forming the cephalic flexure. The mesenchyme covering the ventral surface is compressed and forms cartilage.

The neonate skull and skeletal system is very different to that of the older child or adult. In the adult there are twenty-nine bones in the skull, in a neonate there are approximately thirty-six separate parts.

The occiput is in four parts; the body, squama and two lateral masses or condylar parts. The temporal bone is in two parts, the petrous and the squama. The mastoid is just a bud and will not develop until it is stimulated by the use of the sternocleidomastoid muscle. The sphenoid is in three parts; the body, the greater wing and the lesser wing.

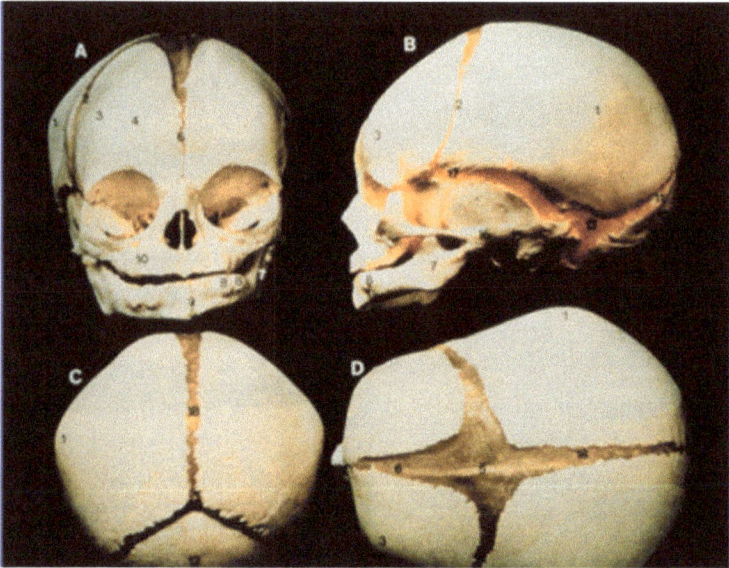

The foetal skull. Notice the small mandibles and the soft sutures and fontanels and the size of the orbits in comparison with the rest of the cranium.

There are six fontanels, which are membranous spacers that allow for growth of the brain and the cranial vault to expand.

The important thing to remember when treating neonates and babies is that they are physically, psychologically and spiritually different from us.

In neonates and very young babies what you feel is unique.

During birth the baby has to absorb the compressive forces as it is pushed down the vaginal canal. Each contraction of the uterus compresses along a cephalo-caudal axis.

Forces are absorbed by the spinal column and the cranial base.

As the birth progresses the chin will flex on to the chest at the same time as being compressed the cervico-thoracic junction tries to accommodate these forces and you get flexion and compression at C7/T1 and T1/T2. This will in turn affect the way the thoracic inlet functions.

The occiput acts as a fulcrum for rotation as it passes the symphysis pubis. If the rotation cannot be accommodated it will resolve on the occipital squama which will affect the lateral masses and the condyles. This is often where cranial base patterns are imparted into the baby.

Neonatal respiration

As the baby is delivered there has to be a change from foetal to neonatal respiration. This first breath is very important.

Before the baby is born the alveoli are filled with fluid and the vascular resistance of the pulmonary circulation is greater than that of the systemic circulation. Blood passes through the ductus arteriosus to the aorta thus bypassing the lungs.

All this has to change. The fluid in the lungs is slowly absorbed into the vasculature and the lymphatics. Altered haemodynamics, and a decrease in body temperature associated with an increase of carbon dioxide and a decrease of oxygen, demands that the neonate takes its first breath. The lungs will expand as an air fluid interface develops.

The surface tension within the alveoli is decreased by the presence of surfactant.

Surfactant is a phospholipid combined with protein and it is secreted into the alveolar space. It decreases the surface tension, which prevents the elastic tendency of the lung parenchyma pulling the alveoli together thus preventing expansion.

According to Dr Jane Carreiro, surfactant also has a role in maintaining the patency of the small airways and also within the immune system increasing phagocytic activity in pulmonary macrophages.

As the first breath is taken the muscles of respiration begin to work. The main muscles of respiration are the scalene muscle, quadratus lumborum muscle and the intercostal muscles. The intercostal muscles are formed as the diaphragm descends and the primitive rib cartilage condenses.

The external intercostal muscles are the muscles of inspiration and the internal intercostal muscles the muscles of expiration. To allow these muscles to work effectively the scalene muscle anchors and elevates the first rib by contracting, this allows the external intercostal muscles to contract sequentially and thus elevate the ribs superiorly. Conversely the quadratus lumborum muscle contracts and fixes the lower ribs in conjunction with the oblique abdominal muscles. This allows the internal intercostal muscles to contract sequentially pulling the ribs downwards.

The rectus abdominus and the transversus abdominus, along with the oblique abdominal muscles, all assist respiration and for some time are the primary muscles of expiration by helping to pull the lower ribs downwards.

Finally, the pelvic diaphragm creates a negative pressure within the abdominal and thoracic cavity and the hip flexors are called in to assist in times of respiratory distress.

In addition to this there is no cough reflex in a new-born. The pharynx is a tube anchored posteriorly by the pharyngeal raphe, which is suspended from the inferior surface of the sphenoid and the petrous temporal bones. In inhalation the musculature tends to collapse. To support inhalation the genioglossus muscle contracts taking the tongue anteriorly, which has the effect of opening the posterior pharyngeal space. The vocal chords also abduct to decrease the laryngeal resistance.

During breathing the abdominal viscera act as a piston and the diaphragm uses this to lift the ribs and expand the size of the rib cage. Infants rely on abdominal breathing.

Diagnosis and observation takes time. As we progress in our career as an osteopath, we have to be patient and realise that our skills take a long time to develop. We cannot rush them. So, take your time, be comfortable with yourself and your ability.

Sutherland said, "Take time in making your assessment and diagnosis. Often it will be the second or may be the third visit before you can make a complete assessment and diagnosis."

The first thing you do when parents and their baby present in your practice is to observe the parents, especially the mother.

Look at her pelvis and sacrum, discretely.

What type of pelvis does she have? Is the pelvic bowl wide or is it narrow or android? Does the sacrum have a normal curve or is it flat, is it convex? The shape of the sacrum will make a big difference in the way the foetus travels down the vaginal canal. The shape and mobility of the pelvis can determine whether the birth was going to be easy or more difficult. If the sacrum is flat or convex then as the baby passes down the canal sweeping past the sacrum the face will be dragged downwards and the child will have similar problems to that of a face presentation.

The parents' interaction with the baby is also important to observe. Are they relaxed, are they tense or anxious are they irritated? Are they comfortable with the child?

I remember one set of parents at the school clinic who simply dumped the baby in the middle of the plinth and each parent sat in opposite corners of the room. The students were quite shocked and when they asked the parents if they would they would pick the baby up and hold it the mother looked at the father and said, "you wanted it, you hold it."

The relationship between the parents and the child is so important and especially as the child gets older. The first seven years of its life are extremely important. What the child will be like in the rest of their life is on the whole mapped out in those first seven years.

History taking

Good history taking is essential.

Although the majority of this chapter is aimed at neonates and babies, I feel that at this point I should explain that when taking a case history of and older child when they can interact always put your questions to the child.

It is the child that is the patient and although they may in the end only offer very little and you will have to say, "Shall we ask mummy/daddy?" But by following this procedure you are involving them in what is often a rather difficult time.

The following are guidelines as to the questions you should ask.

"Why have you brought your baby to see me?"

A seemingly simple question but often parents of become a little confused as to the specific problem, so let them talk and then gently bring them round to answering specific questions.

"Is it the first, second or third child?"

Often the second and third labour is easier than the first although the baby can descend the canal quite quickly which does not allow for moulding to take place. Fourth and fifth babies are often delivered very quickly.

What is the maternal age?

Nowadays we are seeing many mothers who have their first babies in their mid to late thirties and even early forties.

However, you do see babies who have very young mothers who often do not have a lot of support. I remember one young mother who came into our practice and was seen by my French colleague Gaelle. The mother was sixteen years old and when she asked the mother why she had a baby at such a young age the mother replied that she wanted something to love.

You have to be prepared for every eventuality in practice and be objective, caring and a good listener, and not be judgemental.

You carry on building a picture.

Was the pregnancy planned or unplanned?

Often when the pregnancy is unplanned there is an element of shock within the baby (shock will be described later in this chapter.)

How was the mother during the pregnancy?

Was she content, frightened, was it a good pregnancy?

Were there any physical or mental traumas?

Traumas especially mental ones can have quite an effect on the foetus. Whatever happens to the mother will affect the foetus?

If there is bereavement or if their partner has left them during the pregnancy, it will not only have a profound effect on the mother, but also on the foetus. These are babies that often do not sleep and are very fractious. The membrane is very tight and when you just touch or lift the baby, not palpating in any depth, it will feel very tense. There is no softness in the tissues, no calmness and the baby often feels quite rigid. When you apply touch, the baby reacts and does not want to be touched.

Did the mother have a bleed at any time?

I remember a seeing a baby which only slept for short periods of time and any noise or movement was enough to wake it. The parents were at the end of their tether, having had very little sleep. On examination the membrane was very tight and tense, exhibiting all the signs that I call shock within the system.

The parents gave a history of a good pregnancy; the mother was happy and there were no events that caused her distress.

Except, she quietly confided that she had a bleed at ten weeks. It was a heavy bleed and she thought she had lost the baby, but a scan revealed that it was still there. I asked her about the bleed and I came to the conclusion that during that bleed she probably lost a baby, the twin of the one I was seeing. Hence why the baby was so stressed; it had lost its twin.

I treated the baby and talked a lot to the parents and after a few weeks he was sleeping well and the parents much more relaxed.

It can be quite traumatic for the mother if she feels that she could miscarry and therefore an element of shock or anxiety is transferred to the foetus.

Is the mother on any medication?

Some drugs can be transferred to the baby via the mother's milk, which can affect the baby in the way it sleeps and behaves, particularly in the case of anti-epileptic drugs. I had another mother with a very fractious baby that did not respond well to treatment and as I knew she was epileptic I suggested she consulted her doctor to try to get her medication changed. The doctor called me and asked why I had suggested this, I explained everything to her and that I had read that the medication the patient was on could be transferred to the baby via her breast milk. The doctor changed the medication and the baby improved dramatically.

Did the pregnancy go to term or was it premature or overdue?

When did the head engage?

Or didn't it?

How long was the labour?

How long was the final stage and what medication was given?

Was there any intervention such as forceps or ventouse suction?

Was the baby breach at any time?

Did the mother have a caesarean section?

There are always more questions you can ask. Take the time to explore fully and always listen carefully to the parents' responses. Gradually you will develop the skill of moving them on and getting the answers to the right questions.

You need to know how long after the birth was the umbilical cord cut. I find this quite important as often the cord is cut whilst it is still pulsating and I feel this gives backlash to the gut and the abdomen. When this happens, the baby is more prone to having difficulty passing stools.

What was the first cry like, good or weak?

This is important for the expansion of the lungs and the changes that occur within the heart and the major vessels. The foramen ovale becomes closes by apposition of the septum as the pressure between the atria become equal, and the obliteration of the ductus arteriosus although being gradual begins at birth and eventually become the ligament arteriosum.

Observation

Observation is paramount when examining the baby or child.

Does it look well? Is it attentive, does it move its limbs well, are the eyes bright, does it react to stimulus?

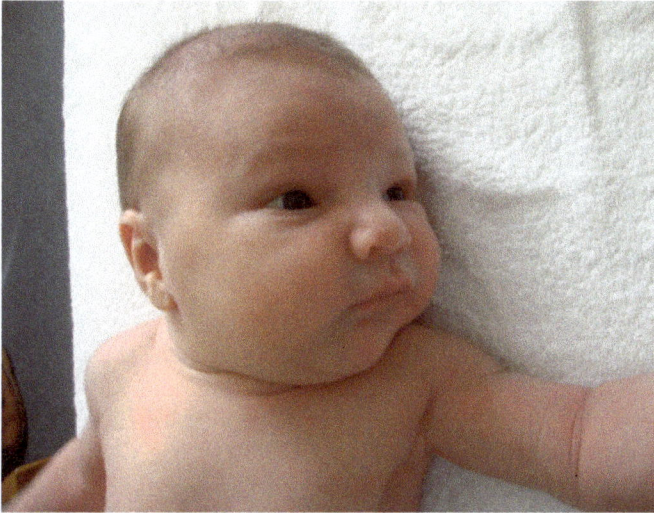

Is the child aware of things and what is happening around it? Now look at the eyes; does it focus and follow?

Are there signs of jaundice, what is the tone of the skin?

What colour is the skin, are there signs of poor venous drainage?

Does the baby frown? This could be a sign of compression from the sphenobasilar symphysis, or where the frontal has been pushed downwards and is compressed, affecting the structures of the naso/oropharynx causing the baby to have some nasal congestion or the baby might snore.

Babies who present having had the head engaged in the pelvic bowl for some time prior to the birth, anything from one to five weeks, will tend to present with a head that is flatter, the vault bones are very soft developed in membrane. The parietals, occiput and frontals are pushed down caudally. When this occurs, you must consider what is happening to the sagittal sinus. This is where the arachnoid granulations are situated, where some of the cerebrospinal fluid (CSF) is reabsorbed. The new-born infant needs a good flow of CSF and a good blood supply, so you have to consider ways of lifting the parietals and therefore the falx, the sagittal sinus and the sinus membranous system.

The opposite of this is when babies are delivered very quickly without a period of restitution. These babies will often present with elongated heads where the parietals bones and the occiput and frontals are lifted up cranially and look like the shape of a bishop's mitre. This also often happens where ventouse suction has been applied to assist the birth.

Think of the anatomy.

What is happening to the vault bones and the membrane? The membrane will have become elevated, taking with it the ethmoid, the falx and the tentorium and the cranial base within the cranium and as the membrane travels down the neural canal all structures associated with it will also be lifted cranially, as will the sacrum. Palpation of the sacrum will reveal that it is very high, and pulled upwards out of the soft pelvic bowl. This elevation will also affect the respiratory diaphragm causing it to be very domed and tight. Breathing can be compromised and these are the babies that hiccup a lot.

Continue your observation and look to see if there are any obvious signs of cranial base patterns? These base patterns are important and give you a good indication as to how the body is functioning.

Patterns are schematic representations that were invented by Dr Sutherland, according to Dr Anne Wales. The point of reference for these patterns is the sphenobasilar synchondrosis.

There are two types of strain patterns:
Physiological strains – torsion, side bending rotation and compression, and non-physiological strains – vertical and lateral strains.

Torsion is when the sphenoid and the occiput rotate in opposite directions on an anterior-posterior axis, usually in response to a compression of the peripheral articulations in one quadrant. They are named by the superior wing of the sphenoid.

Side bending rotation happens when the sphenoid and occiput rotate in opposite directions on a vertical axis and in the same direction on the anteroposterior axis. This results in excessive pressure on one side of the head. They are named after the convex side.

Compression is a lesion where the basisphenoid and the basilar part of the occiput have been approximated so that motion is impaired, either moderately or where motion is completely lost. This is induced by powerful uterine contractions especially where there is severe resistance or trauma.

Vertical strain is when the sphenoid moves in flexion and the occiput moves into extension or vice versa.

Lateral strain is where the sphenoid and the occiput rotate in the same direction around a parallel vertical axis. Forceps delivery may induce lateral strains.

Observe the shape of the face and the body. Does it favour one side more than the other? Are the eyes the same shape? What is happening to the maxilla? Remember the maxilla is very short and squat in a baby.

Observation of the maxilla will tell you how the sphenoid is moving. As discussed previously the sphenoid has no direct relationship with the maxillae and movement is transferred from the sphenoid to the maxillae via the zygoma, palatines and the vomer, normally termed the speed reducers.

Visual observation gives you a very good idea of what is happening within the body.

Does the child breathe into the abdomen? Do the eyes focus? Does the baby/child hear well?

If it is an older child how does it relate to the parents? Is it very active, even hyperactive? Does it do what it is told? Is it shy?

131

All these things are important when trying to build up a picture.

Remember this is integrated osteopathy and we are looking at the psyche as well as the viscera and the musculoskeletal system.

If the child is older, how is the co-ordination? How are they walking/crawling? How does the spine move when they are crawling? What is the attention span like?

When I evaluate by palpation, I always have the baby on a pillow, held on the knees between the parent and myself. This has several advantages.

Firstly, it is far better than placing a tiny infant on a large plinth and by using the pillow you have constant eye contact with the parent and the parent has contact with the baby. Remember that the baby is very precious and the parents are probably sceptical about what you are doing and often very wary of another person touching their new baby.

Always explain to them what you are doing and why. Explain your examination and the anatomy. I remember a neurosurgeon telling us at a postgraduate course that he always explained everything to the patient and family. He said they probably only took in ten per cent of what he told them, but they appreciated that he had taken the time to talk them through what was going to happen.

Good communication is so important in practice.

Do it in terms that they can understand and it will give them confidence and a greater understanding as to what you will be trying to achieve. The parents want to know what your findings are and what you are attempting to do and at the end of the session you must be in a position to deliver a treatment plan.

Continue your examination by undressing the baby/child and continue to observe. If the child is older, always explain to them what you require and ask for their agreement. It is very simple to communicate, you can even make a game of it. You are including the child in the decision process and even at a very young age, this is important.

Is there symmetry? Are the extremities symmetrical or does one foot, one arm externally rotate more than the other? Is the chest symmetrical, is one side more pronounced with the ribs moving better on one side more than the other, allowing the lung on one side to be slightly compromised?

Does the baby have problems with the feet such as Talipes equinovarus, which is due to compression in utero? This often resolves spontaneously or with exercises that you can give the parents to do. I find this works extremely well and most mothers and fathers are very happy to exercise the foot into external rotation whilst sitting at home in the evening.

When you have completed your visual examination, you can then move on to evaluating musculoskeletal structure and the involuntary mechanism.

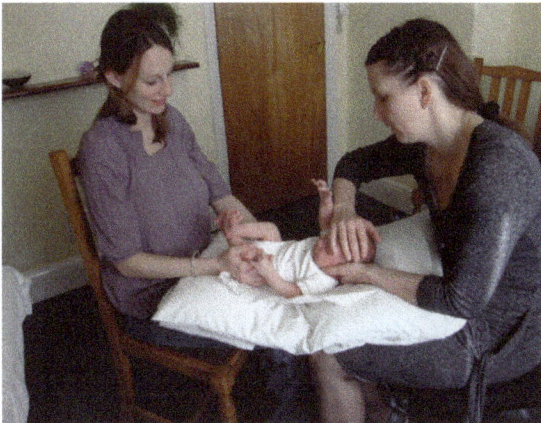

Have the baby on a pillow between you and the parent.

Another advantage of having the baby on a pillow is that when you wish to move from the sacrum and thorax, you can simply rotate the pillow with the baby still lying on it.

During the examination, I explain the anatomy of the new-born, the make-up of the cranium and the difference between the cranial base and the vault to the parents. The explanation continues by showing that there has to be a firm base from which the cranial vault can rapidly expand in size. I tell them that a foetal head resembles a soft-boiled egg filled with porridge.

I talk about the membrane, how it encapsulates the brain and the spinal cord, often showing them pictures and drawings and that it looks like a large tadpole with the sacrum attached to the membrane at the lower end.

Finally, I explain that the sacrum and the pelvis are all in small pieces held in what are like jiffy bags of membrane.

All of this goes a long way in getting the parents to understand that what you are doing when treating their baby is based on a deep knowledge of applied anatomy and physiology.

When palpating the involuntary mechanism (IVM) in a young baby or a neonate use soft, gentle hands.

First, put your hands on the baby and feel the tissue tone. Is it soft and pliable or is it tense and tight? Build a picture of how this body is operating.

I always begin by palpating the lower leg and especially the fibula. This strange, twisted bone will give you a very good indication of what the mechanism is doing in the flexion and extension phases. Do they externally rotate simultaneously in the flexion phase and is the movement the same for each side?

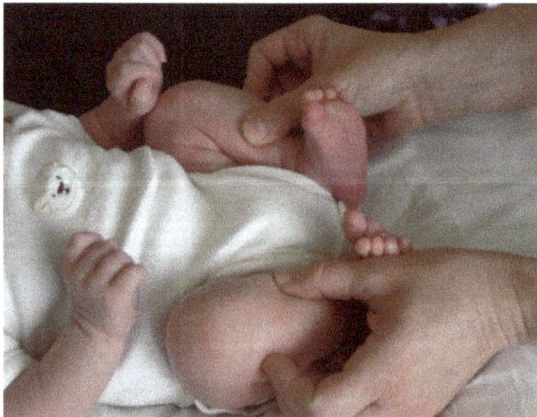

Palpation of the fibula.

When you have done this, move your hands up and palpate the hip joints to ascertain if there are any undue clicks within the joint when taking it into circumduction.

Place one hand under the hip in contact with the hip joint and the pelvic floor. Place the knee in the palm of your other hand and your index finger along the shaft of the femur, with the rest of the fingers holding the flexor muscles and your thumb in contact with the extensor muscles. With a gentle but firm downward pressure, compress the hip and take it into circumduction. Palpate for any "clicks" or quick changes in movement. Most clicks you feel will be soft membranous clicks, however if you feel a distinct hard click then further investigation has to be undertaken, usually by ultrasound. as the head of the femur might not be engaging in the infantile acetabulum and the baby could have a congenitally dislocating hip.

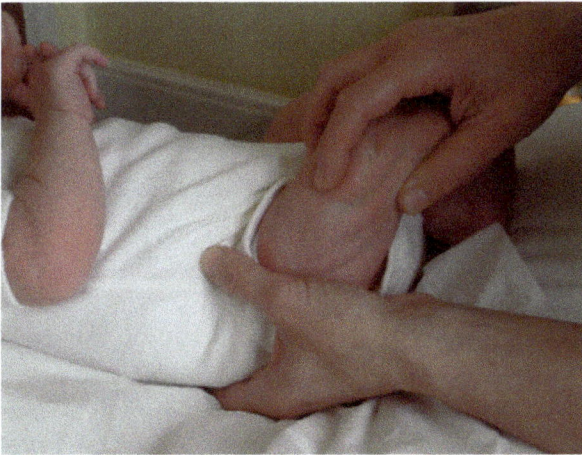

Palpating for irregularities in the hip joint.

Continue your examination of the pelvis and sacrum. Place the palm of your hands under both hip joints. Your fingers of each hand should spread out towards the spine. The sacrum should be under your ring finger and little finger whilst the middle and index fingers are resting on the lumbar spine and the thoraco-lumbar junction.

Now your thumbs will be in a position to lie across what will become the anterior superior iliac spine.

With this simple hold you will have the whole pelvis in your hands. You will feel the small pelvic bones externally and internally rotating as the sacrum moves from flexion to extension.

You will now be in the best position to palpate and assess the sacrum. Does it breathe, does it float, and does it feel soft or hard? Is it compressed or is it elevated? How it is seated in the pelvis?

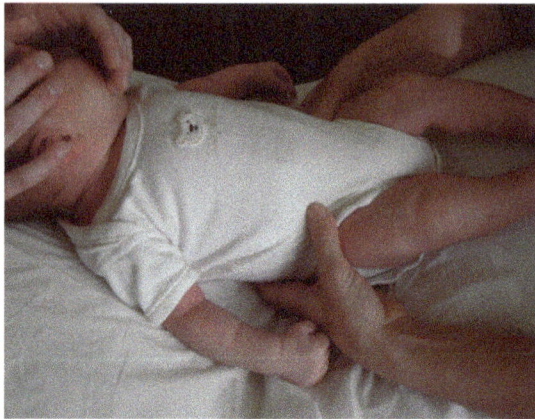

Hand hold for palpating and balancing the sacrum.

Balancing the Sacrum

Using this hold you can balance the sacrum in the midline using the membrane and by taking the constituent parts of the pelvis into whichever lesion it needs to go.

Follow the movement.

You will often find that it will begin to move in one direction on one side and then movement will begin on the other side often simultaneously. You have to be like a juggler keeping all the balls in the air, because you have to concentrate on the midline at the same time as following the lesion. The sacrum will tend to swing and somewhere in this movement you will find a fulcrum. Balance all the movement around this fulcrum gradually refining it until it is perfectly balanced. When you reach this point, you will feel everything soften.

I sometimes think it is as though the tissue "sighs".

From the sacrum it is easy to move your hands cranially to palpate the diaphragm. This can be done in a number of ways.

If you are right handed, place your left hand on the dorsal surface and using your ventral hand place the middle finger on the xiphoid sternum and spread your index finger, ring finger and little finger around the twelfth rib and contact the diaphragm. Use your ventral fingers like the spokes of an umbrella and palpate between your hands from the midline laterally.

The second method is to have the dorsal hand as above and the ventral horizontally across the diaphragm. With this hold you will be palpating with the ring and little finger and the hypothenar eminence. Again, feel between your hands.

When evaluating the diaphragm, look to see if it is elevated or compressed caudally. Does it feel soft; are the crura tight or relaxed? Remember the structures that pass through the diaphragm. Fifty per cent of the lymph drainage goes through the diaphragm, as do a number of major vessels.

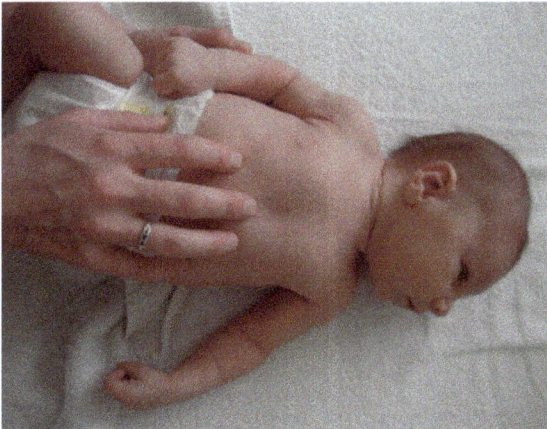

Palpation of the diaphragm.

From the diaphragm you can easily move to examine the dorsal spine.

To assess the dorsal spine, place your hands either side under the baby so that your fingers are in touch with the spinous processes and the erector spinae.

Palpate the expression of the IVM.

Watch how the spine will shorten in the flexion phase and elongate in the extension phase.

Does it feel comfortable? Can you palpate any areas where the movement is restricted or excessively mobile?

You will find areas of restriction often from the compression associated with the birth process. Each of these restrictions can be balanced individually allowing for better mobility of the spine.

Using the same hold evaluate the ribs individually for each side and if necessary, balance them using balanced ligamentous techniques.

Dr Jane Carreiro reported in An Osteopathic approach to children 2003 that osteopathic observation of 1,600 neonates immediately after birth demonstrated the presence of a functional fulcrum in the deep tissues at the level of T3-T4 on the right. She continued to say that since this fulcrum was only observed in new-borns who attempted spontaneous breathing, it is presumed to be associated with the transition to air breathing.

Tissue strains at the area of this fulcrum have been found in older children with chronic respiratory diseases.

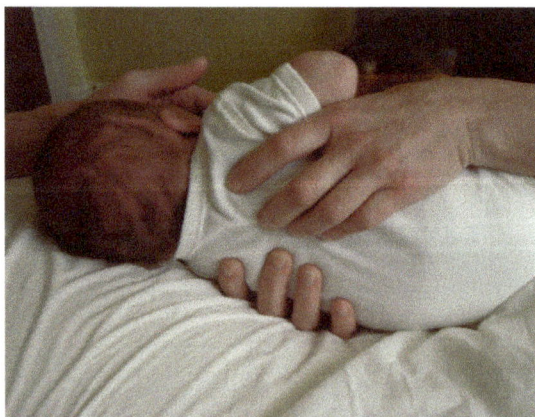

Palpation of the thoracic spine.

Another method for doing this is to cradle the baby on your forearm, one hand in between the legs and the chest and abdomen resting on the forearm. This is a really good way of evaluating the ribs, dorsal spine and the cranial vault. You can easily slide your hand up the thoracic spine and onto the vault of the cranium. Spread your hand and you will be in contact with the parietal bones, the occiput and the frontal bones. This method is especially and effective when the baby is fractious and unsettled. By gentle rocking the baby tends to settle more and this makes life much easier for you.

I find that babies being held this way often relax, especially if they have colic and I think that this is because the stomach and the gut can hang down with gravity and this effect tends to ease the stress on the structures.

Using this hold you will be able to balance all the ribs and the thoracic spine and then you can move to the cranial vault.

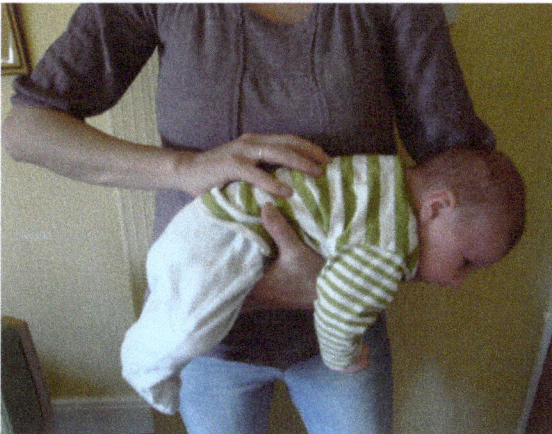

Balancing the ribs with baby lying prone along your arm.

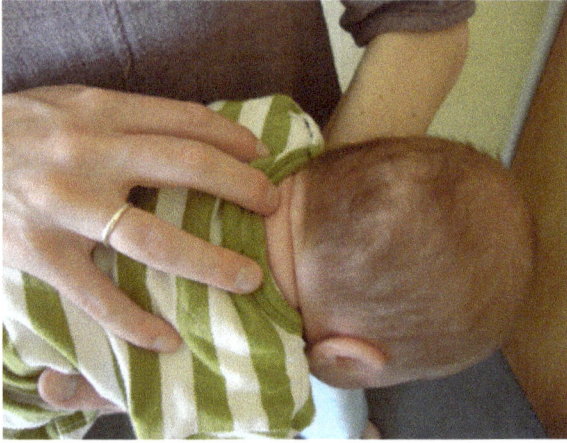

Middle finger on spinous process, index finger and ring finger balancing the upper ribs.

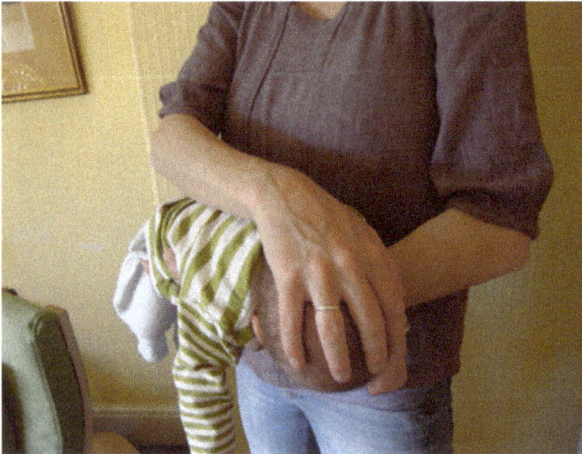

The hand can easily move onto the cranium, middle finger on the falx cerebri and the index and ring fingers either side contacting the membrane. From this position you can easily balance he membrane around the sella turcica.

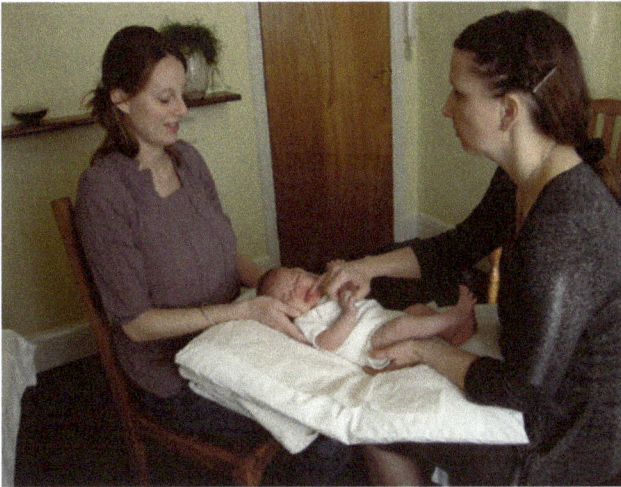

Now you can cast your attention to the thoracic inlet and the cranium.

The thoracic inlet takes on several changes throughout the birth process. At one point during the birth, the chin flexes onto the chest and causes compression of the inlet.

Osteopaths have for years regarded the thoracic inlet as a very important area. When you consider the complexity of this area you begin to understand its importance.

There are a large number of lymph nodes in what is termed the anterior triangle. This is the area between the tip of the mandible and the clavicles, which underlies the platysma and forms part of the thoracic inlet.

The clavicle forms the inferior border and the movement, or more to the point the lack of movement, can affect the lymphatic drainage. The brachial plexus and subclavian vessels also pass through this inlet.

The attachment for the sterno-clavicular joint has fascial links with that of the hyoid and with a band running laterally connects with the thoracic inlet structures.

Caroline Stone, in her article in the Osteopath (1999) states that Sibson's fascia is a name given to a fascial/connective tissue sheet which attaches to the internal edge of the first rib, and passes medially to the deep cervical fascia and covers the dome of the parietal pleura as it does so. As Caroline states, Sibson's fascia is a disputed structure, which is often accredited other names, however it does seem to be a separate structure to the endothoracic fascia and the parietal pleura and can be reinforced by one or other of the scalene muscles.

Barral (1991) states that irritation in the parietal pleura and upper lobe of the lung can affect the mechanics of the lower cervical spine.

I always palpate the cranium last, why? Because I want to get a really good idea of how this body is working before I place my hands on the cranium which some babies find very sensitive or even intrusive.

When you begin palpating be gentle, and yet be positive. There are no sutures and the only joint within the skull is the atlantooccipital joint. The vault is formed in membrane and the cranial bones are sleeved in pockets of membrane and periosteum. The cranial base is formed in cartilage, which forms a good foundation for the skull to grow as the brain grows.

The periosteum and the dura are one and the same as they invaginate where they meet at the edges of the bony structures. Each vault bone is held within a pocket of membrane and is therefore very pliable and easy to move them.

As previously stated, there are six fontanelles which act as spacers allowing the skull to accommodate growth. The fontanelles at anion, pterion and inion usually close at six to eight weeks, but the anterior fontanelle does not fuse for up to eighteen months.

In this chapter I feel it is important to recap some of the techniques I would use when treating neonates and babies.

The Parietal Lift

The parietals are comparatively large and firmly attached to the membrane. They have to be lifted in the *extension phase*. In the flexion stage the parietal bones are moving inferiorly and laterally and therefore it not possible to lift them and if you try all you will succeed in doing is compounding the problem. To lift them you either use one hand or the fingers of both hands depending on the size of your hands and the child's head. As you lift them you will find them rising. *Be careful to lift symmetrically.* When they reach the top of the lift you will feel them hanging loosely (wobbling); wait and soon you will feel them returning. *Do not let them go.*

Gently let them settle back in position. In doing so firstly you will find it feels very different and secondly you will have altered the cranial base. Because the membrane is attached around the foramen magnum by lifting the parietals you will have reshaped the foramen. This will have a big effect on the whole mechanism. Also, by doing so you will have altered the shape and given space to the sagittal sinus. This is very important because in babies who have experienced a difficult birth, especially those where the foetal head was engaged in the pelvic bowl two to three weeks prior to birth often have a flat vault thus compressing the sagittal sinus and therefore there will be altered venous flow and the arachnoid granulations will be compromised as will the reabsorption of CSF.

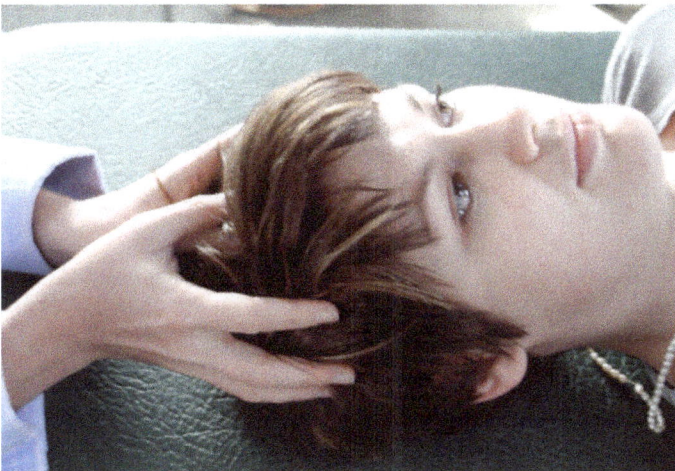

The parietal lift hold.

The Frontal Lift

The naso/oropharynx in a baby or infant is quite complex. You will find many instances of babies presenting with nasal congestion, breathing through the mouth. When visually examining the baby, you will notice a frown where the frontal has been pushed downwards in utero. It is important you remember the anatomy of this area. Remember how soft this bone will be and its relationship of the ethmoid within the frontal notch and the lesser wing of the sphenoid, the greater wing of the sphenoid as well as that with the zygoma and the other speed reducers, the vomer and the palatine will be compromised.

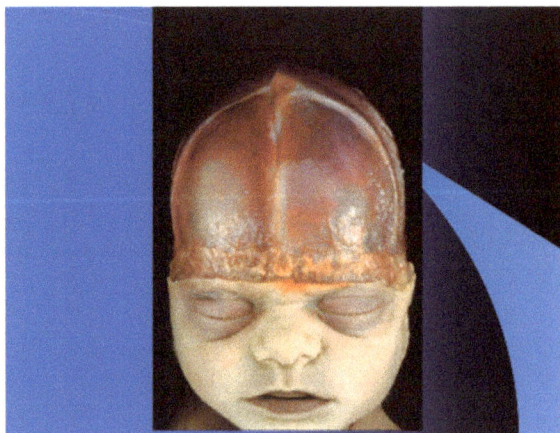

Neonate frontal bone showing the metopic and coronal sutures.
With kind permission of the Willard/Carreiro Collection

It is therefore important to restore proper mobility within this area and to begin with you would have to lift the frontal bone to enable it to move freely and reduce the compression that it will have on the other structures related to it.

Place one hand under the occiput and the other hand transversely across the frontal (see Fig 5.)

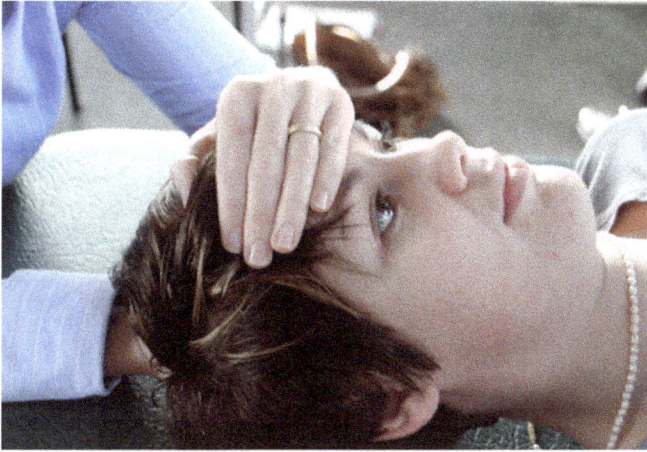

Fig 5 the frontal lift.

This is a direct technique so once started you must complete the procedure.

Think between your hands. You have the membrane in your hands and going anteroposteriorly from the internal occipital protuberance to the crystagali is the falx cerebri. Using the fourth and fifth fingers you lift the frontal in the extension phase, you literally suck it up.

You will find that the frontal will lift off easily and you take it superiorly and slightly anteriorly as far as it will go. When you reach the extreme of the movement you may feel it wobble slightly, wait. When it is ready it will begin to return slowly, follow it and as you get to the point where it is settling back in position try to exaggerate the width to attempt to widen the ethmoidal notch. In this way you will be able to influence the movement in the nasopharynx.

Let the mechanism return to a normal pattern and come off.

Decompression of the cranial base

During a normal vaginal birth, the baby has to absorb a considerable amount of compression as the uterus contracts pushing the baby further down the birth canal. This mechanical compression is seen mainly at the sacrum, the thoracic spine and ribs, the thoracic inlet and the basiocciput and the cranial base.

There is only one joint in the neonate cranium and that is the atlanto- occipital joint. This is often compressed during the birth and due to the softness of the occiput changes can occur that introduce patterns within the skull.

The neonate occiput is in four parts, the body, the squama and the two condylar parts or lateral masses, as they are sometimes known. The condyles are shaped to sit on the atlas and looking from the anterior part of the bone they go posterior, laterally and inferiorly.

The four parts of the occiput are tethered by strong ligamentous and membranous tissue. Using the following technique, the practitioner can decompress and balance the cranial base.

To do this you have to engage the membrane.

Once you have done this find the falx cerebri and follow it to the straight sinus. Remember this is where the falx cerebri, the tentorium and the falx cerebelli coalesce. Now palpate the falx cerebelli that runs from the inferior border of the straight sinus inferiorly and slightly anteriorly to the edge of the foramen magnum. In the technique to decompress the cranial base this will be one of your focal points.

Now move your hands under the cranium.

Your fifth digits (little fingers) should be as close together as you can get them and as far down towards the cranial base as you can. The little fingers should be in contact with the falx cerebelli. I.e. in the midline.

Your ring finger should now be able to slide under the cranial base and engage the lateral masses. In neonates and babies, before the basiocciput fuses, the occiput is in four distinct parts, and the lateral masses that become condyles are floating separately in pockets of membrane.

With the ring fingers of both hands now engage the lateral masses.

You now need to concentrate on your ring fingers and little fingers at the same time. With your ring fingers gently disengage the body of the occiput via the falx cerebelli. Note it is not traction, but just a simple disengagement. You have to be positive and firm in your approach. As you disengage the body of the occiput you will feel the lateral masses begin to move, follow them into their lesion patterns and eventually you will find a fulcrum about which you can balance the two lateral masses. If at any time you feel that the movement has stopped or slows right down just increase the distraction with your little fingers and movement will return. You will be giving yourself more space.

When the two masses become balanced you will feel the whole cranial base soften and expand, as though it melts. When this occurs, you have completed the technique.

Treating a neonate allows you the unique facility to balance the membrane using the anterior dural girdle. The anterior dural girdle is better known as the lesser wing of the sphenoid bone and for the first five to six weeks of life the lesser wing is in membrane although the sphenoid being part of the cranial base is mainly formed in cartilage.

The fact that the lesser wing of the sphenoid is in membrane can be used to our advantage. It enables us to balance the complete membrane and have a pronounced effect on the foramen magnum and the cranial base.

It should also be remembered that at this age the crista galli of the ethmoid is much more posterior and therefore the attachment of the falx cerebri is also further posterior towards the sella turcica and the diaphragm of selle.

The anterior dural girdle forms an important part of the dural membrane in conjunction with the tentorium and the falx cerebri. There are now five separate girdles that can be balanced, the two separate parts of the anterior dural girdle [lesser wing of the sphenoid] which will become the right and left lesser wings of the sphenoid, the two tentoria, left and right and the falx cerebelli.

These five components can be balanced around a fulcrum in the midline in the area of the diaphragm of selle, roughly around the infundibulum.

This can be accomplished with the baby supine, lying on a pillow between me and the parent, you can use the tips of your fingers of both hands or just have one hand on the vault and the other cradling the cranial base.

Then balance all the components around your fulcrum.

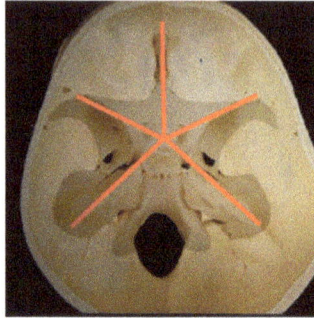

I cannot leave this chapter without considering infantile colic.

Infantile colic presents at around two to three weeks after the birth and can last up to four months.

The most common cause of infantile colic is lactose intolerance, a survey at St Georges Hospital London.

Dr Jane Carreiro states (Osteopathic approach to children) that based on osteopathic structural findings, most children presenting with colic fall into one of three groups. Functional gastrointestinal disturbance, persistent nociceptive or painful stimuli and some combination of the two.

Carreiro also states that colic often coincides with the early development of the neck muscles leading to a mechanical strain. Visceral somatic reflexes in the mid and lower thoracic spine also has an effect.

She also states that the common osteopathic view of colic is that the effect of these strains on the vagus nerve which may contribute to vagal irritation by compressing the nerves vaso nervosum.

Gut motility and function are immature in the neonate This leads to increased transit times and immature hormone and enzyme function thus promoting the production of internal gasses.

Vagal and parasympathetic influences on the gut act to increase tonic contractions and the lack of mature innervation patterns in the gut wall gives rise to uncoordinated contractions rather than a peristaltic wave.

Osteopathic treatment focused on the areas of dysfunction have been found to aid the baby whist a more mature system develops.

Developmental milestones

Whilst observing the baby/child you have to consider if it is reaching its developmental milestones.

Table of Developmental Milestones courtesy of Dr Jane Carreiro

	Reflexes	Gross Motor	Fine Motor	Social	Language
NB	Rooting, sucking, moro	Grasp, closed fist, flexion	Follow to midline	Regards face	
4th week	Atonic neck reflex	Loss of involuntary grasp	Follows past midline	Smiles responsively	Responds to bell
2 Mo		Lifts head 90* head steady	Opens fist Hands together	Smiles spontaneously	Squeals, early vocalisation
4 Mo	Head righting	Raises chest, rolls over loss of head lag	Reaches, regards	laughing	Turns to voice
6 Mo	Protective equilibrium	Bears some weight on legs, sits, creeps	Rakes, takes 2 cubes, trans between hands	Seeks partially hidden toy, peekaboo, self feeds crackers	babbles

	Reflexes	Gross Motor	Fine Motor	Social	Language
8 Mo	parachute	Pulls self up, sits by self, crawls	Bangs cubes together	Pat a cake, shy with strangers	Intonational patterns
10 Mo		Cruises, stands	Points, pincer grasp	Plays ball throws	Dada/ mamma specific
12 Mo		Walks, stoops	approximates	Indicates want uses cup	3 words body part
18 Mo		Steps, kicks ball, throws	Scribble, tower of 4 cubes	Imitation play, uses spoon, undresses	Combines 2 words, names pictures
2 Yr		Jumps, lifts one foot for 1 second	8 cubes imitates line	Help dress, wash and dries hands	Can "show me" 2 step commands
3 Yr		Tricycle	Copies circle	Buttons, dresses with supervision	Cold, thirsty, hungry, colour opposites
4 Yr		Hops, catch ball, heel to toe walk	3 body parts Imitates square	Separates from mother	Exaggeration opp., defines

www.ingramcontent.com/pod-product-compliance
Lightning Source LLC
Chambersburg PA
CBHW042117190326
41519CB00030B/7527